Working with Attachment Trauma

The Adult Attachment Projective Picture System (AAP) has served as a prominent assessment tool for adults and adolescents internationally for over 20 years. This book introduces the AAP and illustrates the powerful potential for implementing the AAP in clinical practice for assessment, client conceptualization, treatment planning, analysis, and as a therapeutic guide.

Chapters discuss the full scope of incomplete pathological mourning for attachment trauma, including for the first time in the field Failure to Mourn and Preoccupation with Personal Suffering. Seasoned clinical researchers and psychotherapists provide a snapshot of their clients' unique attachment characteristics and defensive exclusion strategies as assessed by the AAP, and discuss how to use this information in treatment, as well as how to present the AAP results to their clients.

This book introduces readers to how the AAP can be used with adolescents, adults, and couples, and in custody evaluation and foster care.

Carol George, Ph.D., is an internationally renowned attachment expert and provides extensive teaching and consultation in the clinical application of attachment. Her books include the *Adult Attachment Projective Picture System*, *Attachment Disorganization*, and *Disorganized Attachment and Caregiving*.

Julie Wargo Aikins, Ph.D., is an expert in developmental psychopathology and parent-child relationships and consults on the clinical application of attachment theory. She conducts research that includes various measures of attachment, writes and presents on attachment theory, and trains on the use of the Adult Attachment Projective Picture System.

Melissa Lehmann, Ph.D., is a clinical psychologist at the Center for Therapeutic Assessment. Her practice involves assessment and therapy with clients who have experienced attachment trauma, as well as providing consultation to other clinicians in this area.

"The editors have brought together an impressive group of international researchers and practitioners to highlight the clinical use of the Adult Attachment Projective Picture System (AAP). The chapters offer compelling examples of the AAP's value for clinical practice, assessment, or intervention, especially in the context of attachment trauma and intergenerational transmission risk. It is a must for any student or practitioner working with vulnerable adults and parents and seeking to understand the fundamental underlying attachment mechanisms involved in the development of trauma and resilience."

Chantal Cyr, Ph.D., *Full professor, Department of Psychology, Université du Québec à Montréal, and Canada Research Chair in Child Attachment and Development*

"This book is a milestone in demonstrating the broad applicability and critical value of the AAP. The creativity and clinical acumen of the authors will benefit a host of future clients. Moreover, this book builds a bridge from assessors to therapists who will be well-served to have attachment patterns assessed in troubled clients. Kudos to the authors for such a valuable contribution!"

Hale Martin, Ph.D., *Clinical Professor, University of Denver, Therapeutic Assessment Institute*

"This book is a must-have resource for anyone using or considering using the AAP, and anyone interested in assessing attachment. Initial chapters provide an orientation to the foundation for the task stimuli and how responses to them are classified, its uses in practice, and a review of the neurophysiological correlates of its scores. In the remaining chapters, talented experts illustrate the illuminating and unique information emerging from the AAP across a range of ages, settings, and presenting issues."

Gregory J. Meyer, Ph.D., *Professor, University of Toledo; former Editor of* Journal of Personality Assessment

"The Adult Attachment Projective Picture System (AAP) is an invaluable tool for assessment in medical settings to help clients consider the role of developmentally-based psychodynamic processes in their presenting problems. This book expands the scope of the AAP deep into practice with sophisticated and moving case studies that describe the diversity of contexts in which the AAP can enhance clinical insight and facilitate therapeutic dialogue."

David J. York, Ph.D., *Psychological Assessment and Testing Service, Christiana Care Health System, Newark, Delaware*

Working with Attachment Trauma

Clinical Application of the Adult Attachment Projective Picture System

Edited by
Carol George
Julie Wargo Aikins
Melissa Lehmann

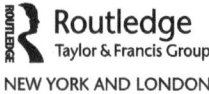
Routledge
Taylor & Francis Group

NEW YORK AND LONDON

Designed cover image: © Getty Images

First published 2023
by Routledge
605 Third Avenue, New York, NY 10158

and by Routledge
4 Park Square, Milton Park, Abingdon, Oxon, OX14 4RN

Routledge is an imprint of the Taylor & Francis Group, an informa business

ISBN: 978-1-032-10461-4 (hbk)
ISBN: 978-1-032-10460-7 (pbk)
ISBN: 978-1-003-21543-1 (ebk)

DOI: 10.4324/9781003215431

Typeset in Sabon
by codeMantra

To Malcolm West, 1942–2020

Contents

Editors

Carol George, Ph.D., is Professor Emerita of Psychology and Distinguished Research Fellow at Mills College in Oakland, CA. She received her doctorate in developmental psychology from the University of California, Berkeley, in 1984. She developed the Adult Attachment Projective Picture System (AAP) with Malcolm West, Ph.D., which is becoming one of the most clinically used attachment measures in assessment communities such as Therapeutic Assessment and the Society for Personality Assessment. Dr. George is an internationally renowned attachment expert and teaches courses and trainings in attachment theory and assessment. Dr. George has collaborated on developing the most attachment assessments in her field, including the *Attachment Doll Play Assessment* for children aged 4–11, the *Adult Attachment Interview,* the *Caregiving Interview,* and the *Caregiving Helplessness Questionnaire.* She has authored numerous papers and book chapters on adult and child attachment and parental caregiving. In addition to the seminal AAP volume, her books include *Attachment Disorganization* and *Disorganized Attachment and Caregiving* with Dr. Judith Solomon. She is Assistant Editor on the editorial board of *Attachment and Human Development.* She does extensive consultation in the clinical application of attachment and developmental psychopathology, integrating attachment in treatment for professionals working with clients across the life span.

Julie Wargo Aikins, Ph.D., is an Associate Professor at Merrill Palmer Skillman Institute and the Department of Psychiatry and Behavioral Neuroscience at Wayne State University in Detroit, MI. She received her doctorate in child clinical psychology from The Pennsylvania State University in 1999. Dr. Wargo Aikins has examined the influence of parents and parent-child relationships on child adjustment among children ranging from preschool through the adolescent years. She has been using the Adult Attachment Projective Picture System in her research for the last 20 years to examine topics such as attachment stability and change, attachment representations within Active Duty and Veteran military populations, and attachment representations within families impacted by stress and change. Dr. Wargo Aikins is a member of the International Adult Attachment Projective Picture System Training Consortium. She has trained many clinicians and research colleagues on the use and coding of the AAP and does consultation regarding the clinical application of the AAP.

Melissa Lehmann, Ph.D., is a Licensed Psychologist in private practice at the Center for Therapeutic Assessment in Austin, Texas. She received her degree in counseling psychology from the University of Texas at Austin in 2008, where she became focused on Therapeutic Assessment and attachment theory. Her dissertation research used the Adult Attachment Projective Picture System (AAP) in a study of juvenile sex offenders. She is a founding member of the Therapeutic Assessment Institute and also a member of the International Adult Attachment Projective Picture System Training Consortium. She consults and trains clinical professionals internationally. Dr. Lehmann's clinical work uses the AAP in conjunction with other personality measures in Therapeutic Assessments with adults, adolescents, and families. Her expertise includes using the AAP in psychotherapy for clients with childhood attachment trauma. Dr. Lehmann has presented numerous AAP workshops and seminars on the use of the AAP in Therapeutic Assessment.

Contributors

Marie Achille, Ph.D., Department of Psychology, Université de Montréal, Montréal, Canada. Dr. Achille studied psychology at McGill (B.Sc.) and Simon Fraser University (M.A., Ph.D.), and completed a post-doctoral fellowship at the Stanford University Behavioral Medicine Clinic. She began her career as a clinical psychologist, caring for patients and living donors before and after transplantation. She is now a professor of psychology at Université de Montréal. Her research interests focus on psychosocial issues around solid organ transplantation, living donation, and the ethics of consent to donation.

Deane E. Aikins, Ph.D., John D. Dingell VA Medical Center, Department of Psychiatry and Behavioral Neuroscience, Associate Professor of Psychology, Wayne State University, Detroit, MI. Dr. Aikins is a psychologist and researcher at the John D. Dingle VA Medical Healthcare Center in Detroit, Michigan. He is an associate professor at Wayne State University in the Department of Psychiatry and Behavioral Neuroscience. Dr. Aikins is an expert in military stress, risk, and resilience factors. He engages in both clinical work and research in Active Duty and Veteran populations.

Marie-Julie Béliveau, Ph.D., Department of Psychology and the Infant Psychology Clinic, Université de Montréal, Montréal, Canada, and Hôpital Rivière-des-Prairies, Montréal, Canada. Dr. Béliveau is a clinical psychologist and professor of psychology at Université de Montréal. She studied psychology at Concordia University (B.A.) and Université du Québec à Montréal (M. Ps., Ph.D.). Her graduate studies focused on mother-child attachment in early childhood and maternal attachment representations, for which she was trained in AAP coding. She worked as a developmental psychologist in child psychiatry and is now teaching and supervising child and adolescent assessment to graduate students. Her current line of research focuses on diagnostic issues, parental perceptions of child problems and adaptation of clinical children.

Anna Buchheim, Ph.D., Professor of Psychology, University of Innsbruck, Innsbruck, Austria. Dr. Buchheim is a licensed psychologist and psychoanalyst (IPA). She graduated from the University of Ulm, where she completed her dissertation, habilitation, and Psychoanalytic Training. She is currently a Full Professor for Clinical Psychology and Vice Rector for Human Resources at the University of Innsbruck. Her research focuses on clinical attachment, intergenerational transmission of attachment, psychotherapy research, and neuroscience of human attachment. Dr. Buchheim is the certified AAP trainer for the German speaking countries in the AAP Training Consortium.

Livia Buratta, Ph.D., Department of Philosophy, Social Sciences, and Education, University of Perugia, Perugia, Italy. Dr. Buratta is Adjunct Professor at the University of Perugia where she teaches Elements of Psychodynamic Psychology in the Department of Philosophy, Social Sciences and Education. She also collaborates with the Psychological Unit of the Healthy Lifestyle Institute (C.U.R.I.A.Mo. - University of Perugia).

Alex Clark, D. Clinical Psychology, Clinical Psychologist, Cornwall Partnership NHS Trust, Cornwall, England. Dr. Clark is a clinical psychologist within Children and Adolescent Mental Health Services for people with intellectual disabilities in Cornwall Partnership NHS Trust (UK). Alex obtained his doctorate in clinical psychology from the University of Plymouth.

Rex Collins, Ph.D., The Willow Centre, Toronto, Canada. Dr. Collins is a Psychologist and Clinical Director of the Willow Centre in Toronto, a private clinic which provides assessment and treatment for infants, children, adolescents, and their families. He has a longstanding interest in assessing and treating adolescents, drawing from ten years on the Adolescent Inpatient Unit at Sunnybrook Health Sciences Hospital in Toronto. He is a graduate of the Toronto Child Psychotherapy Program and is a passionate advocate for the use of projective techniques in psychological assessment, in particular the Rorschach.

Elisa Delvecchio, Ph.D., Department of Philosophy, Social Sciences, and Education, University of Perugia, Perugia, Italy. Dr. Delvecchio is Associate Professor of Psychology at the University of Perugia (Italy). She is the coordinator of the "Psychology and Cultures Lab" at the International Human-being Research Centre. She is involved in international and national projects aimed to promote psychological wellbeing and inclusion of vulnerable groups. She is a certified AAP trainer in the Italian language in the AAP Training Consortium.

Daniela Di Riso, Ph.D., Department of Developmental Psychology and Socialization, University of Padova, Padova, Italy. Dr. Di Riso is a

Psychologist, Psychotherapist and Associate Professor of Clinical and Dynamic Psychology at the University of Padova. She practices at the clinical service of psychological counseling for university students (SAP-CP) at SCUP.

Stephen E. Finn, Ph.D., Clinical Psychologist, Center for the Therapeutic Assessment, Austin, TX. Dr. Finn is a licensed psychologist at the Center for Therapeutic Assessment in Austin, Texas, where he is also Clinical Associate Professor of Psychology at the University of Texas at Austin. Dr. Finn is best known for helping to develop Therapeutic Assessment, a semi-structured model of collaborative psychological assessment, where tests are used as "empathy magnifiers" to help clients address persistent problems in living. Dr. Finn helped found the Therapeutic Assessment Institute, the European Center for Therapeutic Assessment in Milan, Italy, and the Asian-Pacific Center for Therapeutic Assessment in Tokyo, Japan.

Deanna Gallichan, D. Clinical Psychology, Consultant Clinical Psychologist, Livewell Southwest CIC, Plymouth, England. Dr. Gallichan works as a consultant clinical psychologist within an NHS funded service for people with intellectual disabilities in Plymouth, Devon, UK. Deanna obtained her Ph.D. from the University of Birmingham and her doctorate in clinical psychology from the University of Exeter.

Manuela Gander, Ph.D., Postdoctoral Fellow, Department of Child and Adolescent Psychiatry, Medical University of Innsbruck, Innsbruck, Austria. Dr. Gander is a licensed clinical psychologist. She graduated from the University of Innsbruck, where she completed her dissertation and habilitation in the field of developmental and clinical psychology. She works as a senior lecturer at the Institute of Psychology at the University of Innsbruck and as a clinical psychologist at the Child and Adolescent Psychiatry in Innsbruck. Her research focuses on the role of attachment for the onset, course and outcome of adolescents with mental disorders, neurophysiological correlates of attachment and attachment related interventions. Dr. Gander is a certified AAP judge and co-trainer for the German speaking countries.

David Joubert, Ph.D., Associate Professor of Criminology, University of Ottawa, Ottawa, Canada. Dr. Joubert is a psychologist and member of the Ordre des Psychologues du Québec since 2008. He graduated from the Université du Québec à Montréal in clinical psychology and in applied criminology from the University of Ottawa. He is currently Associate Professor of Criminology at the University of Ottawa and Clinical Psychologist at the Y2 Clinic in Gatineau. His research interests include assessment and intervention in forensic settings, risk and personality assessment, mental health problems in prison settings, and attachment in children and adults.

Katie Kivisto, Ph.D., Associate Professor of Clinical Psychology, University of Indianapolis, Indianapolis, IN. Dr. Kivisto is an Associate Professor in Clinical Child Psychology at the University of Indianapolis. She teaches courses in human development, child psychopathology, and interventions with youth and families. Her perspective on development is deeply rooted in attachment theory, and especially how foundational attachment relationships influence life-long emotion regulation, adjustment, and relationships. She is an Indiana licensed psychologist working with children, adolescents, and adults.

Steffani Kizziar, Psy.D., Portland Mental Health and Wellness, Portland, OR. Dr. Kizziar is a post-doctoral resident. She holds a master's degree in Infant Mental Health from Mills College (Oakland, CA) and a master's and doctorate in Clinical Psychology from University of Indianapolis. She serves adolescents, adults, and couples from an attachment-informed, psychodynamic perspective.

Caroline Lee, Psy.D., is a licensed psychologist in private practice in Dallas, TX. Caroline received her degree in Clinical Psychology from Rosemead School of Psychology in Los Angeles, CA. She completed her internship at the Institute of Living in Hartford, CT and trained in Therapeutic Assessment during her fellowship year. Caroline uses the AAP clinically in her private practice in Dallas, TX, where she conducts Therapeutic Assessments with adolescents and adults. She also codes AAPs for professionals from around the world and trains other clinicians in this particular measure.

Marie Leblond, Ph.D., Department of Psychology, Université de Montréal, Montréal, Canada. Dr. Leblond studied psychology at University of Trois-Rivieres and Paris Descartes (B.Sc.) and completed a Ph.D. in clinical psychology, specialized in childhood and adolescence, at the University of Montreal. She works at the Douglas Mental Institute, Montreal, where she treats adolescents with eating disorders. Her main areas of research are identity development and parental attitudes in adolescents with renal chronic diseases.

Adriana Lis, Psy.D., Department of Developmental Psychology and Socialization, University of Padova, Padova, Italy. Dr. Lis is Full Professor of Clinical Psychology at the University of Padova. She has authored many papers on attachment and the AAP. Dr. Lis is an Honorary member of the AIP, Associazione Italiana di Psicologia. She is a certified AAP trainer in the Italian language in the AAP Training Consortium.

Claudia Mazzeschi, Ph.D., Department of Philosophy, Social Sciences, and Education, University of Perugia, Perugia, Italy. Dr. Mazzeschi is a Psychoanalyst and Psychotherapist and Full Professor of Clinical and Dynamic Psychology at the University of Perugia. She is President of the Master Course Degree in Assessment of Individual Functioning in Clinical and Health Psychology, Scientific Director and Coordinator of the Psychological Unit of the Healthy Lifestyle Institute (C.U.R.I.A.Mo.- University of Perugia), where she also coordinates the clinical services. She is a certified AAP trainer in the Italian language in the AAP Training Consortium.

Ashley Petersen, Psy.D., Clinical Psychologist, Jennifer E. Manfre & Associates, Woodbridge, IL. Dr. Petersen is a clinical psychologist and Associate Professor of Psychology at Illinois Institute of Technology. She graduated from the California School of Professional Psychology. She currently provides clinical and neuropsychological assessment at a private practice. Her interests include assessment, attachment, trauma, and cognitive behavioral therapy.

Michael Poulakis, Psy.D., Assistant Professor of Clinical Psychology, University of Indianapolis, Indianapolis, IN. Dr. Poulakis is an Assistant Professor at the University of Indianapolis, College of Applied Behavioral Sciences. He immigrated to the United States from Greece and received his doctorate from the University of Indianapolis. He teaches undergraduate and graduate courses. His research lab at UINDY focuses on diversity, addictions, South Asian psychology, and LGBTQ issues. His research expertise is consensual qualitative methodology.

Nancy Poulter, D. Clinical Psychology, Clinical Psychologist, Cornwall Partnership NHS Trust, Cornwell, England. Dr. Poulter is a clinical psychologist within both the Adult and Children and Adolescent Mental Health Services for people with intellectual disabilities in Cornwall Partnership NHS Trust (UK). Nancy obtained her doctorate in clinical psychology from the University of Plymouth.

Silvia Salcuni, Ph.D., Department of Developmental Psychology and Socialization, University of Padova, Padova, Italy. Dr. Salcuni is Psychologist, Psychotherapist, and an Associate Professor in Psychodynamic Psychology at the University of Padova. Dr. Salcuni coordinates the clinical service of psychological counseling for university students (SAP-CP) at SCUP. She teaches Adult Psychological Assessment in the Bachelor degree and Clinical Evaluation and Treatment for child and adolescent Master degree programs at the School of Psychology at University of Padova.

Talia B. Shafir, Ph.D., Psycho-Physical Therapist, Private Practice, New York, NY. Dr. Shafir practices Somatic and Spiritual Psychology. She is a Registered Somatic Movement Educator-Therapist and Clinical Hypnotherapist specializing in psychophysical approaches to trauma and adult attachment. She is the author of *Bridging the Trauma-Adult Attachment Connection Through Somatic Movement (Journal of Body Movement and Dance in Psychotherapy)*.

Kate Stoneman, D. Clinical Psychology, Clinical Psychologist, Cornwall Partnership NHS Trust, Cornwall, England. Dr. Stoneman is a clinical psychologist within Children and Adolescent Mental Health Services for people with intellectual disabilities in Cornwall Partnership NHS Trust (UK). Dr. Stoneman obtained her doctorate in clinical psychology from the University of Plymouth.

Linda Webster, Ph.D., Professor of Education and Senior Associate Dean, Bernerd School of Education, University of the Pacific, Stockton, CA. Dr. Webster is professor emerita at the University of the Pacific in the Counseling Psychology Department. She earned her Ph.D. from UC Berkeley in Human Development and worked as a licensed psychologist for eight years with a county mental health clinic before entering academia. Her research has focused on the measurement and treatment of attachment trauma in children and adolescents. She currently works part-time at the Center for Psychotherapy in Antioch, CA, specializing in assessment and therapy with children and adolescents who have experienced developmental trauma.

Preface

The Adult Attachment Projective Picture System (AAP) has come of age since its debut in the field of attachment assessment a little over 20 years ago. Malcolm West's original goal when he started on the AAP path was to create a practical developmentally based assessment of attachment that adhered to the Bowlby-Ainsworth theory of attachment. "Mac" was an old-school psychoanalyst privy to the power of projective assessments (now often termed free-response measures) to tap processes and sensitivities that are too easily "edited out" of conscious-driven self-report measures. He was also a scientist who endorsed the value of validity and reliability in test development. Dabbling with the original stimuli in 1994, Mac brought Carol George on board as an expert collaborator whose background extended from attachment assessment with infants using the *Strange Situation* (Ainsworth et al., 1978) to adulthood using the *Adult Attachment Interview* (George et al., 1984), as well as parenting assessments and children's projective doll play. As a result, the AAP they co-created became more nuanced and applicable than previous adult attachment measures and was well received when they trained their first group of professionals in 1999.

The nuances of attachment are difficult to capture. Attachment theory emphasizes the development of the self in the context of biologically based relationships, beginning with the infant's first relationship with attachment figures. How we think about ourselves as worthy of care and our attachment figures as trustworthy to provide that care has a finger in every aspect of our relationships and mental health. The AAP uncovers not only our thinking about questions relating to the attachment relationship but also our views of balance and connectedness in relationships with others in our lives.

One of the most important contributors to mental health is how we manage experiences of attachment trauma. Attachment trauma is poorly defined in the field, to date, primarily adhering to a life events approach such as labeling trauma as loss or maltreatment. This narrow approach restricts our work as clinicians and researchers and fails to capture the complexity of individuals' experiences. Clients come into our rooms puzzled by why they feel such pain and distress when their experiences do not adhere to the list of events found on a trauma schedule. The position we adopt here is that attachment trauma includes all experiences where our attachment figures failed to protect us (George & Solomon, 2008; Solomon & George, 1996). Because many clients understand attachment trauma as confined to loss or abuse, we find they cannot describe why they are in such emotional pain, often thinking that their feelings are "irrational" or unwarranted. A crucial component of the AAP is to uncover the affective underpinnings that clinicians can explore with their clients as failed protection and attachment trauma. Clients report that using the AAP to help them "name" trauma is validating and reduces their shame.

Trauma must be mourned (Bowlby, 1980). A unique feature of the AAP is the identification of the three forms of incomplete pathological mourning that Bowlby stressed in his writings as assaults to mental health. In addition to the well-known Unresolved mourning group, the AAP identifies Failed Mourning and Preoccupation with Personal Suffering. Just like therapeutic approaches differ depending on clients' designation as secure or insecure, the therapeutic starting points will be better realized from knowing individuals' forms of pathological mourning.

This book is written by clinicians and researchers who apply the AAP to their work. There is a vast repertoire of academic papers and books that provide readers with the details of attachment theory and generalized examples of its utility in the clinical sphere. This book is intended to be a clinician's first introduction to using the AAP as a clinical tool. We assume the reader knows the basics of attachment theory. Our goal is to introduce for the first time in the field a toolbox that shows the versatility of using the AAP with adults, adolescents, and parents. The clinicians contributing to this book are seasoned AAP users. In addition to describing their clients, we asked them to address many of the stickier issues in attachment assessment that are unaddressed in other writings, for example, how to use the AAP to think about intervention recommendations or psychotherapy or how to discuss the results of the AAP assessment with clients or their caregivers.

The book is organized into four sections. The first section provides basic AAP background. The first chapter provides an overview of how the assessment scoring and classification work. The second chapter describes how clinicians who use the AAP have responded to the measure. The third chapter describes the comprehensive use of the AAP in mental health research with adults and adolescents, including a glimpse of the extensive work these authors have done using the AAP in neurophysiological settings. The second section focuses on attachment trauma and pathological mourning, focusing first on how the basic scoring system is expanded to identify Failed Mourning, Preoccupation with Personal Suffering, and Unresolved trauma. The other three chapters in this section focus specifically on assessment and treatment of clients in these groups. The third section presents a range of cases using the AAP in adult assessment and psychotherapy. They include, for example, addressing the utility of using the AAP to document progress and attachment representational change over time and the embodiment of attachment trauma and application of the AAP with somatic therapy. Other chapters describe using the AAP in psychoanalytic psychotherapy and with adults with intellectual disabilities. The fourth section provides examples of using the AAP in a broad range of settings with adolescents, from foster care to hospital and medical clinic settings such as kidney transplant or obesity. Two chapters in this section use the AAP to try to unravel the complexities of adolescent psychopathology and show how the AAP adds a deeper understanding of diagnoses and interventions than typical psychiatric approaches.

The AAP delves deeply into attachment. Our clients and research participants are so much more than a classification group. We thank our contributors for demonstrating how the AAP provides a personal fingerprint of each client and unveils their unique defensive processing and self-representations. We hope that these chapters will show how the AAP helps us achieve Bowlby's goals in assessment and psychotherapy, to provide a secure base where our clients can explore and think about the deficits and disappointments in their attachment lives.

In as much as this book introduces clinical application, it is not a primer in AAP scoring. More details, including other case studies, are described in the first AAP book (George & West, 2012). We encourage our readers to follow our work, and our workshops and trainings. Updates on these events are found on our website www.attachmentprojective.com.

References

Ainsworth, M. D. S., Blehar, M., Waters, E., & Wall, S. (1978). *Patterns of attachment: A psychological study of the strange situation*. Erlbaum.

George, C., Kaplan, N., & Main, M. (1984). *The adult attachment interview* [Unpublished interview]. University of California, Berkeley.

George, C., & Solomon, J. (2008). The caregiving system: A behavioral systems approach to parenting. In J. Cassidy & P. R. Shaver (Eds.), *Handbook of attachment: Theory, research, and clinical applications* (2nd ed., pp. 833–856). Guilford Press.

George, C., & West, M. (2012). *The adult attachment projective picture system: Attachment theory and assessment in adults*. Guilford Press.

Solomon, J., & George, C. (1996). Defining the caregiving system: Toward a theory of caregiving. *Infant Mental Health Journal*, 17(3), 183–197. https://doi.org/0.1002/(SICI)1097-0355(199623)17:3<198::AID-IMHJ2>3.0.CO;2-L

Part 1
Foundations

Part I

Foundations

1 The Adult Attachment Projective Picture System

Assessing attachment in adults and adolescents

Carol George

Historically, attachment has been in the domain of developmental psychologists mainly concerned with the study of the role of individual differences in attachment in normative development. Its rise to influence in clinical psychology and contribution to psychotherapy is consonant with John Bowlby's original goal for attachment theory as a foundational construct for understanding personality functioning, relationship problems, psychological distress, and psychopathology across the life span (Ainsworth, 1989; Bowlby, 1982, 1988). Attachment theory is compatible with all clinical assessment and treatment approaches that consider childhood experiences an important contributor to adolescent and adult functioning (e.g., Buchheim et al., 2013; Herrmann et al., 2018; Slade, 2016).

Clinical application of attachment constructs requires clarity about the differences between developmental representational measures of adult attachment and social-cognitive evaluations of attachment style. Developmental representational measures of adult attachment assess attachment status, which describes patterns of thinking and the effects of childhood attachment experiences. Attachment style is a social-cognitive personality construct. Its conceptualization and assessments measure attachment in terms of two personality dimensions, avoidance vs. anxiety or positive vs. negative self, which is essentially a reinterpretation of Millon's (1969) model of personality (Bartholomew & Horowitz, 1999). The original endeavor of attachment style was to investigate the roots of loneliness based on readers' responses to a three-item questionnaire published in popular commercial magazines (Hazan & Shaver, 1987). The content domain of attachment style assessments is limited to traits derived from empirical factor analyses of adults' responses to questions about relationships with romantic partners (beginning with college students' long-term dating) rather than the developmental and ethological principles Bowlby (1982) deemed essential to attachment theory. The expansive discussion of Bowlby's conceptual underpinnings that is now applied to attachment style was added retrospectively after these measures had been developed. Following the Bowlby-Ainsworth tradition, developmental attachment measures emphasize the importance of

DOI: 10.4324/9781003215431-2

assessment that activates the attachment system in order to "see attachment in action" (i.e., attachment activating contexts). By contrast, the attachment style approach asks individuals to report generically on their feelings in relationships; attachment is never observed in action. Further, attachment style theorists extrapolated this model from being a model of romantic (i.e., sexual system) attachment to building a theory of general human bonding, including coworkers or others not specified by human biology as attachment figures. Therefore, attachment style is a model of human intimate relationships that is more general than the specific relationship Bowlby postulated was central to mental health. Theorists and researchers from these two perspectives agree that these approaches are not isomorphic, even though they both claim to be attachment theory (Crowell et al., 2016; George & West, 2012). The Adult Attachment Projective Picture System (AAP) framework we describe here represents the developmental attachment tradition. Two main strengths of the AAP approach are the evaluation of *unconscious defensive processes* and assessment of *attachment disorganization and trauma* when attachment is activated, which are central to understanding client's interpersonal struggles (George & West, 2012; Solomon & George, 2011a).

The Adult Attachment Interview (AAI, George et al., 1984/1985/1996; Main & Goldwyn, 1985–2003; Main et al., 2003) has been the predominant method used to assess developmental mental representation of adult attachment. The AAI is a semi-structured interview during which individuals are asked to describe past and present relationships with parents and attachment-relevant events during childhood. The interview is subjected to a complex discourse analysis requiring rating on reported experience and current state of mind (discourse style) using 14 nine-point rating scales. From these scales, interviews are judged for the basic four adult attachment categories analogous to children's attachment as assessed using the Strange Situation – Secure-Autonomous, Dismissing, Preoccupied-Enmeshed, and Unresolved. Its validation rests on substantial developmental and clinical research (Bakermans-Kranenburg & van IJzendoorn, 2009).

Despite its strengths, the AAI has significant drawbacks for clinical use. One is its limited assessment scope for attachment trauma. George and West (2012) defined attachment trauma as threats to the integrity of the self or the attachment relationship. The range of attachment trauma experiences clients bring to our practices goes well beyond loss through death or physical and sexual maltreatment, which are the only experiences assessed using the AAI. Another drawback is the AAI's failure to elucidate defensive processes. Defense is core to Bowlby's (1980) thinking and contributes to idiographic and individualized interpretations of our clients' coping strategies. The foundation of AAI classification is derived from philosophical discourse strategies. Except for the few experience rating scales, the AAI scales are not derived from attachment theory.

The practical features of the AAI make it difficult to use in clinical practice. It takes on average one to two hours to administer, and its verbatim transcription and lengthy rating and classification process are difficult to learn, time consuming, cumbersome, and costly. In sum, the AAI poses a significant barrier to clinicians who seek to understand their clients' attachment patterns and relationship difficulties on a deeper level.

The AAP circumvents these clinical and practical problems. This chapter describes how the AAP provides clinicians with a construct valid measure of adult attachment that assesses theoretically derived constructs, defensive processes, and all forms of attachment trauma, including but not limited to maltreatment and loss through death. The practical advantages of the AAP are considerable. The administration time for the AAP is relatively short, and cost-effective coding by reliable judges is available for clinicians who have not achieved reliability. Thus, the AAP is economical and efficient for any clinician who wishes to incorporate attachment theory constructs into their practice and client conceptualizations.

The discussion that follows provides the essential background on the AAP coding and classification system for readers to understand how the AAP assesses attachment and also provides a reference for the AAP case material presented in this volume (see George & West, 2012 for a comprehensive discussion of the AAP). Information regarding training is described at the end of the chapter. Readers are referred to Chapter 2 for a discussion of using the AAP to assess attachment trauma and incomplete pathological mourning, including treatment challenges and general approaches in treatment when mourning is incomplete.

The AAP: Stimulus selection and procedure

The AAP was developed using a construct-oriented approach to create a theory-based set of picture stimuli of individuals in attachment situations. Separation, loss, and fear are the central concepts in attachment theory. Bowlby proposed that being left alone without protection is frightening, whether that be due to a physical separation from an attachment figure or a mental-emotional one, and that being able to manage this fear serves a vital evolutionary function that contributes at every age to mental and biological homeostasis and health (Bowlby, 1973, 1980, 1982).

Picture selection was based on three core elements of attachment theory (Bowlby, 1982). The first, and perhaps most important, is that attachment can only be assessed when the attachment system has been activated. Therefore, scenes were selected that elicit attachment distress depicting the most prominent attachment activators in the Bowlby-Ainsworth approach. These include images portraying potential separation, solitude, death, and fear. The second is variations in the visual portrayal of the accessibility of attachment figures; some stimuli portray individuals alone and others portray individuals in attachment dyads with visible potential attachment figures. Attachment figure perceived availability, combined with responsive and effective care (i.e., sensitivity), defines internal working models of attachment security (Ainsworth et al., 1978; Sroufe et al., 2005). Attachment relationships and regulation are threatened when children feel abandoned and appraise attachment figures as unavailable and failing to provide protection and care (George & Solomon, 2008; Solomon & George, 2011). Infants and young children require attachment figures to be physically present, accessible, and responsive. In adolescence and adulthood, the need and ability to access an attachment figure becomes a "psychological" or representational phenomenon, and AAP patterns demonstrate how representation is an important component of attachment security (Allen, 2008; West & Sheldon-Keller, 1994). The third core concept captured in the AAP pictures is the portrayal of attachment across the life span. Bowlby proposed that attachment is important at every age, from infancy to senescence (Bowlby, 1982, 1973, 1980). AAP scenes depict characters that range in age from children to the elderly.

The AAP begins with a warm-up stimulus. It begins with a warm-up picture of two children playing ball, which is an activity that is neutral concerning attachment and helps clients understand the task. The task then presents individuals with seven attachment stimuli: *Child at Window* (abr. *Window)* – a child looks out a window; *Departure* – an adult man and woman stand facing each other with suitcases positioned nearby; *Bench* – a youth sits alone on a bench; *Bed* – a child and woman sit opposite each other on the child's bed; *Ambulance* – a woman and a child watch ambulance workers load a covered stretcher into an ambulance; *Cemetery* – a man stands by a gravesite headstone; and *Child in Corner* (abr. *Corner)* – a child stands askance in a corner. The stimuli contain only sufficient detail to identify attachment contexts; actions, facial expressions, postures, and background elements are ambiguous. The characters are diverse concerning ethnicity, gender, and age. Examples are provided in Figures 1.1 and 1.2 (see George & West, 2012, for the complete stimulus set and description of stimulus development).

AAP administration takes approximately 30 minutes and is done in a private setting. The administration instructions integrate techniques from traditional elements of free response tasks with semi-structured interviews. In-person administration is preferred. Individuals are given the drawing to hold and asked to describe what is going on in the picture, including what led up to the scene, characters' thoughts or feelings, and the outcome. We recently developed a tele-administration AAP format to use when in-person administration is not possible (David et al., in press, 2021; George et al., 2020)). The responses are audiotaped for transcription and verbatim analysis; transcripts are typically two to three pages in length. Administrators must be trained in administration techniques

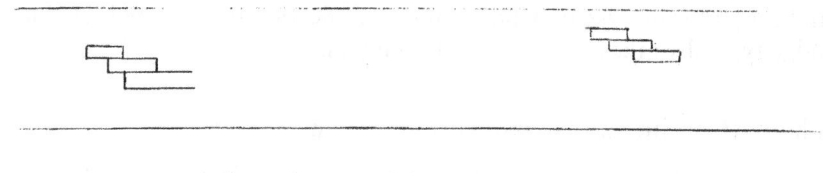

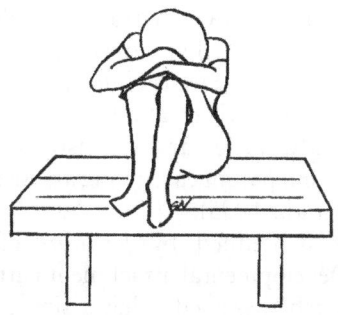

Figure 1.1 Bench *Reproduced with the permission of Carol George.*

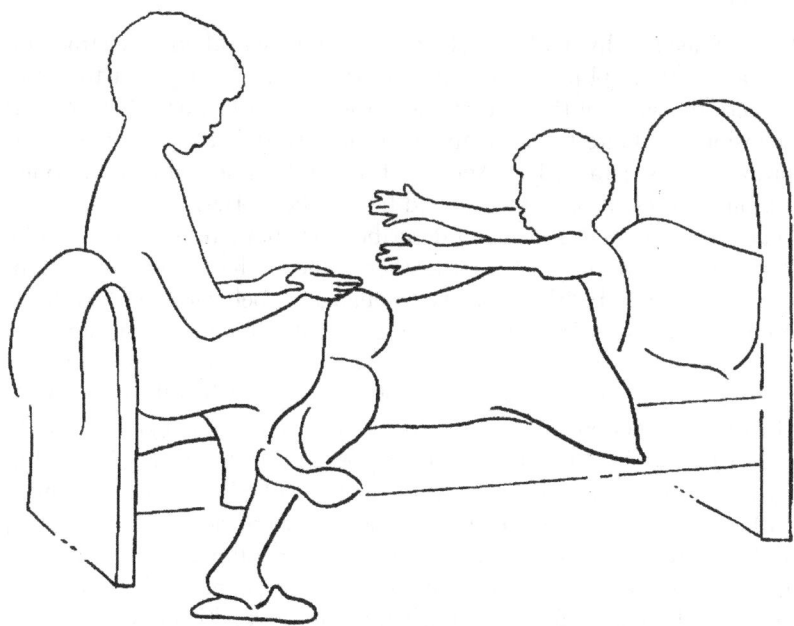

Figure 1.2 Bed *Reproduced with the permission of Carol George.*

but do not need to be attachment experts or trained in the AAP coding and classification system. Coding and classification by a trained reliable judge typically takes about one to two hours.

The AAP coding and classification system

The AAP coding and classification system is the only adult attachment measure that identifies the theoretically defined core attachment constructs following the Bowlby-Ainsworth tradition. The AAP coding scheme integrates salient features that contribute to differentiating patterns of attachment, especially parent-child interaction on reunion in the Strange Situation (Ainsworth et al., 1978; Cassidy & Marvin, 1987–1992; Main & Cassidy, 1988) and defensive processes in child attachment-based doll play and parent caregiving assessments (George & Solomon, 2008; Solomon et al., 1995).

Attachment assessment is defined by *patterns* of responsiveness (Ainsworth et al., 1978). Developmental attachment patterns, in contrast to attachment style, cannot be assessed using a single or paired set of orthogonal dimensions. The AAP system evaluates patterns of responses pertaining to the *story content, defense,* and self-other boundaries in narrative *discourse* (George & West, 2001, 2012; George et al., 1999).

Story content

The AAP asks individuals to tell stories about hypothetical characters. It is not a biographical task, and individuals are not asked to make connections between these stories and their own life story. The content dimensions evaluate the attachment meanings and features of self and relationships (see Table 1.1). Agency of self and connectedness are coded for alone stories; synchrony is coded for dyadic stories.

The *agency of self* dimension describes the character's ability to take constructive steps to address the theme (i.e., what is happening) in the story. Agency is "the capacity to engage in behavior that produces change, the use of relationships to re-establish attachment equilibrium, and/or the capacity to enter and actively explore one's own internal working model" (West & George, 2002, p. 281). It is influenced by an individual's experiences in childhood with attachment figures (Sroufe et al., 2005) and later in life, including psychotherapy or a relationship with a long-term adult partner (Sroufe et al., 2005; Waters & Hamilton, 2000). Agency is required for the "alone" self to preserve integrity (e.g., problem-solving, separation, relationship repair following an argument) and also contributes to maintaining homeostasis, conceived as balanced organized thought and behavior when the individual is flooded by feelings of desperation, helplessness, isolation, fear, or threat.

Table 1.1 Overview of the Adult Attachment Projective System Coding System

Dimension	Stimuli	Definition
Content		
Agency of self	Alone	Story character takes steps to address the situation.
Connectedness	Alone	The story character's desire and ability to be connected to other people.
Synchrony	Dyadic	Reciprocal and mutual attachment–caregiving relationships.
Defense		
Deactivation	All	Shift attention away from attachment; deflect awareness of distress (e.g., authority, social scripts, distance, romance, rejection, neutralize).
Cognitive disconnection	All	Splintered or fractured descriptions of attachment events and emotions (e.g., uncertainty, opposite themes, anxiety, withdrawal, gloss over, shame).
Segregated systems	All	Overwhelmed by frightening and threatening experiences (e.g., helpless, frightened, out of control, isolated, abandoned).
Discourse – self-other boundaries	All	Response includes own life experience in response. Coded as present or absent.

The coding system identifies two levels of *agency of self*. One level, integrated agency refers to the qualities of the integrity of self that are associated with the homeostatic emotion regulation balance and confidence that underpin attachment security (Ainsworth, 1989; Bowlby, 1982; George & Solomon, 2008; Solomon et al., 1995). One form of integrated agency is *haven of safety,* evidenced when the character receives sensitive care from an attachment figure or reaches out to repair or reintegrate a relationship rupture. Another form is *internalized secure base*, a new attachment concept developed for the AAP to capture the capacity for thoughtful self-exploration (George et al., 1999). This concept is a representational interpretation of the secure base phenomenon, which Ainsworth defined as the ability to explore based on the confidence that the attachment figure is available and sensitive to the child's attachment needs (Ainsworth et al., 1978). Attachment representation affords psychological proximity to the attachment figure even in the parent's physical absence (Bowlby, 1982). The internalized secure base refers to that state in which security and self-integrity are derived from the individual's internalized relationship to the attachment figure. It is evidenced in the AAP by themes that describe a character using the solitude portrayed in the alone picture stimuli to explore the thoughts and feelings of their internal world.

A second level of agency reflects the self's capacity to take constructive action in attachment situations, termed *capacity to act*. It is defined as an action that successfully removes the individual from or manages threat, including self-protective behavior, and can occur irrespective of the individual's willingness to think about the source of distress. It is evidenced in the AAP by descriptions of the character engaging in functional or problem-solving behavior.

The *connectedness* dimension evaluates the propensity of the individual to renew or make interpersonal connections in intimate relationships. In addition to attachment relationships, other biologically defined relationships thought to be important in human development include friendships and adult pair bonds. Indeed, Ainsworth and others suggest that these relationships are important sources of emotional support (Ainsworth, 1989; Zeifman & Hazan, 2016). *Connectedness* is evidenced in the AAP when a character who is alone demonstrates the desire and capacity to seek attachment figures, friends, or adult partners. Characters are evaluated as marginally connected when they only seek the help or company of acquaintances or strangers. Characters are not connected when they are blocked from being with others or themes are void of other people, which suggests representations of an alone self that lacks the capacity or desire to seek out others.

Synchrony evaluates whether or not the attachment-caregiving relationships portrayed in the dyadic stimuli are portrayed in a "goal-corrected partnership." Following Bowlby's (1982) discussion of the goal-corrected partnership, *synchrony* is evidenced in dyads by descriptions of reciprocal interaction and demonstrates a commitment to the attachment-caregiving relationship (see also Marvin et al., 2016). The most integrated form of *synchrony* is descriptions of reciprocal interaction depicting dyadic mutual enjoyment or the attachment figure's sensitivity to distress and vulnerability. Functional synchrony does not support balance and homeostasis but helps manage attachment distress from becoming debilitating, even when sensitive reciprocity is not desirable or possible (e.g., the adult explains the situation to the child; a teacher intervenes on the child's behalf). Functional synchrony sometimes entails the attachment figure responding to the situation in a practical way without directly addressing the attachment need (e.g., mother turns on the night light but does not respond directly to the child's cue for a goodnight hug).

Defensive processes

In *Loss*, Bowlby (1980) discussed at length the associations among defense, representation, and affect regulation, and the relation between defensive processes and psychiatric symptoms. His unique approach was to consider defensive processes, a core psychoanalytic concept, from an affective information processing perspective. He viewed defense as a set of automatic unconscious attentional processes that select, exclude, and transform behavior, thought, and emotions to shift attention away from attachment distress and prevent psychological breakdown (see also Hesse & Main, 2006). Bowlby (1980) delineated three forms of defensive exclusion: *deactivation, cognitive disconnection*, and *segregated systems*. Although the importance of defense is acknowledged in the field of attachment (Bretherton & Munholland, 2008; Cassidy & Kobak, 1988; Mikulincer et al., 2009), George and Solomon are the only researchers who have operationally defined and validated Bowlby's approach making it accessible for assessment (George & Solomon, 2008; Solomon et al., 1995). Further, they have shown that identifying an individual's primary defensive strategy is a crucial step to attachment classification; identifying patterns of defensive strategies provides important insight into differences between attachment classification groups and the unique characteristics of individuals with the same classification. Following this work, the AAP identifies Bowlby's three forms of defensive processes. The AAP is the only attachment assessment that provides descriptions of the defenses of adult attachment "in action." Evidence of defensive processing is coded from the words and images produced in the story narrative (see Table 1.1).

Deactivating defenses are defined as shifts in attention away from attachment events, individuals, or feelings. Deactivation deflects and prevents the individual from becoming conscious of attendant attachment distress. Examples of deactivation include emphasis on the importance of following rules, social scripts, achievement and intellect, authority, creating emotional distance, or themes of romance (a diversion of the attachment system to the sexual system). If distress does enter consciousness and characters are described as distressed or in need of care, deactivating defenses produce evaluations of individuals as not deserving care and attachment needs as rejected or neutralized.

Cognitive disconnection was Bowlby's (1980) attempt to modernize the psychoanalytic defense of splitting. Cognitive disconnection breaks apart the elements of attachment from their source, thus undermining consistency and the capability of holding in one's mind a unitary view of events, emotions, and the individuals associated with them. It is evidenced in the AAP by confusion and abrupt representational shifts, oscillations, and sometimes pure confusion. For example, the individual is unable to make decisions about characters or events, sometimes to the point of being inextricably caught between opposing themes (e.g., nighttime or daytime, the girl is happy or sad). Whereas deactivation neutralizes negative affect, disconnection leaks and cannot manage negative affect. Story elements include images of anger or frustration that are dealt with by disconnecting behavior, such as withdrawal, withholding, or attempts to gloss over attachment difficulties in hopes that they will simply go away.

George and Solomon viewed deactivation and cognitive disconnection as normative forms of defense (George & Solomon, 2008; Solomon et al., 1995). "Normative" means that these processes successfully divert attention away from or splinter attachment events, memories, and feelings sufficiently to keep attachment organized. These forms are the primary defensive strategies associated with organized attachment classifications (i.e., Secure, Dismissing, or Preoccupied). Normative defenses can support homeostasis (secure) or at least basic emotional regulation (organized insecure) that helps prevent individuals from becoming flooded and immobilized by the intense levels of fear or threat that disorganize and dysregulate attachment (see Solomon & George, 2011 for review).

Disorganized attachment is associated with Bowlby's (1980) third form of defense, *segregated systems*. The segregated system is defined as an intensified defensive process that locks away the painful "package" of memories and affects associated with threatening attachment experiences from conscious awareness (in information processing terms, working memory). Analogous to the psychoanalytic concept of repression, viewing defense from an information processing perspective provides additional clarity to the process of repression. Segregated systems provide a greater protective shield than the normative exclusion processes of deactivation and cognitive disconnection. Bowlby proposed that activation of these segregated models resulted in such emotional intensity that thought and behavior becomes disorganized and chaotic. When the segregation defense that has been heavily relied upon begins to fail, we may anticipate the breakthrough of traumatic or frightening material. In the AAP, individuals include, for example, descriptions of being afraid, helpless, out of control, or isolated.

Bowlby's approach in defining segregated systems helps us understand more clearly the juxtaposition of signs and symptoms of rigid control, frozen constriction, frightened hypervigilance, over-sensitivity, and dysregulation. It also helps elucidate the psychiatric symptoms of individuals who are classified in the child disorganized-controlling and adult Unresolved attachment groups, especially when their experiences encompass severe abuse or terror (Hesse & Main, 2006; Liotti, 2004; Solomon & George, 2011).

The first coding step is to mark the transcript for evidence of segregated systems. The next step is to evaluate whether the segregated material is reorganized (i.e., managed) in the story response, and the case is judged "resolved" following the nomenclature of the field (Hesse, 2016). Reorganization requires representational management, such as addressing segregated material with agency of self or functional assistance from others. The individual is designated as Unresolved, the AAP group analogous to the AAI Unresolved classification (George & West,

2012; Hesse, 2016), when segregated system material emerges and there is a representational failure to contain the breakthrough.

Discourse: Self-other boundaries

AAP responses are also evaluated for the individual's ability to maintain self-other boundaries while responding to the stimuli. The AAP is not an autobiographical interview. The AAP instructions direct individuals to describe what is happening with hypothetical characters. The "invasion" of material about one's own experience, therefore, demonstrates a failure to maintain the boundaries between self and other during the task and is marked in the transcript as personal experience. This material contributes important information in determining whether the individual's attachment distress is Unresolved; descriptions of one's own frightening or traumatic experiences that are not contained or re-integrated during the response are also indicative of an Unresolved attachment.

Classifications

An attachment classification group is assigned based on an analysis of these coding patterns across the entire set of seven attachment stories.

Secure attachment

The hallmark of attachment security is story responses that demonstrate individuals' abilities and willingness to think about attachment distress or reach out to attachment figures for assistance and comfort. In alone stories, this is demonstrated by elements of the internalized secure base or haven of safety. Many, but not all, secure individuals also demonstrated at the representational level how the integrated agency results in functional behavior, that is, capacity to act (e.g., the girl on the bench thinks about her fight with her parents (internalized secure base) and goes home to talk to them (capacity to act). Their stories about attachment-caregiving relationships in the dyadic stories demonstrate a representational goal-corrected partnership. This can be expressed as caregiver comfort in response to distress or the dyad's mutual enjoyment. Secure transcripts are not "perfect." Integration and mutuality are rarely demonstrated in every story. Rather, the overall pattern of story responses demonstrates the importance and value of connection, integrity of self, and balance in relationships above all other qualities. What is also evident in the AAP coding of a secure individual is how defensive processes are supportive rather than exclusionary. Defensive story elements ultimately help characters integrate attachment affect and events rather than shift attention elsewhere. Secure individuals rarely show blurring of personal experience with hypothetical story boundaries in their responses.

Dismissing attachment

Dismissing attachment is defined by the predominance of deactivating defensive processes without the capacity for integration. The responses typically focus on the facts; emotional details are sparse. This pattern demonstrates the underlying negative self-evaluations, such as being punished or unworthy. Some dismissing responses suggest that individuals appear to understand that integration or sensitivity is important, but they cannot "pull it off" in the story. Digging deeper into the response elements reveals that these attempts are "defensive tricks" (e.g., the man at the gravestone *thinks* about problems he's having at work rather than his relationship with the deceased). Other dismissing responses emphasize attachment situations as challenges amenable to correction by intellectual problem-solving in the absence of relationship sensitivity. For example, attachment figures are portrayed as providing functional care (e.g., goes to school to talk to the boy's teacher instead of comforting the boy), as authoritarian (e.g., a parent makes sure the child understands the rationale for correct behavior), or rejecting (e.g., parent tells the child they are too old for hugs). It follows that the connectedness and synchrony codes typically reflect functional interactions. Blurring personal experience with the hypothetical story is unusual for dismissing individuals, thus demonstrating how a deactivated state of mind maintains strict self-other boundaries.

Preoccupied attachment

Preoccupied attachment is defined by the predominance of cognitive disconnection defensive processes that obscure representations of attachment relationships in the absence of integration. Preoccupied responses typically focus on emotional content; the facts or details of the problems themselves are sparse or ill-defined. The end goal of disconnection is to be happy and not bothered by distress. Responses shift attention away from distress by making the situation or outcome cheery (termed glossing) to prevent having to consciously face negative affect. Preoccupied responses belie the tremendous confusion and mental fog created by disconnecting defenses. Details are offered as fractured descriptions of attachment events (e.g., the married couple is going on vacation or getting a divorce), feelings (e.g., characters could be happy or sad), or by offering two or more completely different story lines. Agency in the alone stories is rare or minimal (e.g., the girl on the bench simply *gets up* rather than going somewhere else). Characters in the alone responses often remain alone, literally disconnected from other people. As with the stories of dismissing individuals, attachment figures may be portrayed as providing functional care (e.g., the grandmother gives the child cookies as they watch the ambulance depart). Attachment figures may also be portrayed as not responding at all, neither sensitive nor rejecting, often because they are too distracted or self-absorbed to notice the child's attachment need. Blurring personal experience with the hypothetical story is quite common in preoccupied responses, demonstrating how difficult it is for preoccupied individuals to maintain self-other boundaries in relationships.

Unresolved attachment

The characteristic quality of Unresolved attachment, as noted in the discussion of classification, is the failure to contain and re-organize stories that evidence segregated system markers. Unresolved responses demonstrate how individuals are flooded by their attachment fears while telling a story and unable to regulate. With the exception of the regulation failure, the story content and the underlying defensive process structure are similar to the other attachment groups.

AAP validity studies

George and West (2012) completed the first AAP validity study. The participants were a culturally diverse community sample of 144 women and men aged 18–72 years (M_{women} = 36.2 years; M_{men} = 26.4 years) living in the United States and Canada. Age, gender, nationality, years of education, verbal intelligence, and social desirability were not related to attachment group classification. The AAP classification match to the AAI was used to evaluate concurrent validity. Interjudge reliability and test-retest reliability over three months were also examined. The AAP-AAI concordance rates for four-group classifications (Secure, Dismissing, Preoccupied, Unresolved) and secure-insecure groups were significant – 90% and 97% classification matches, respectively (all kappas and phis, $p < 0.001$; Pearson's r = 0.84 and 0.88, respectively).

The concordance interjudge reliability rates for three expert judges across all AAP classifications were significant for four-group and secure-insecure classification agreement (all kappas and phis, $p < 0.001$ level; Pearson's r = 0.70–0.89). Test-retest stability from the first testing on a randomly selected subsample of participants was significant (84% stability, kappa and phi, $p < 0.001$; Pearson's r = 0.70, $p < 0.001$).

Several other AAP-AAI concordance studies with other samples have demonstrated strong interjudge and classification concordances with kappas at $p < 0.001$ levels (e.g., Buchheim & George, 2011; Buchheim et al., 2018). One study did not report satisfactory classification concordance (Jones-Mason et al., 2015). Three expert judges reviewed the AAPs in this study. They reported that the major problem that likely contributed to the poor concordance was incomplete AAP administration. This study demonstrated how incorrect administration and the failure to follow instructions for probing will result in inadequate story material to make valid classifications. In response to the COVID pandemic of 2020–2021, a virtual administration method was developed to use with clients who were not able to attend in-person assessment sessions. This method was recently validated for clinical use (David et al., in press, 2021).

A comprehensive discussion of basic and clinical research using the AAP with adults and adolescents is beyond the scope of this chapter. Citations and abstracts of studies and clinical applications are available on the AAP website (www.attachmentprojective.com). To highlight, the AAP has been used in a range of studies and applications, including parenting and children's adjustment and developmental risk (e.g., Béliveau & Moss, 2005; Cyr et al., 2003) and divorce-related custody evaluation (e.g., Isaacs et al., 2011), the correlates of Unresolved attachment (Fitzke et al., 2013; Gander et al., 2020; Joubert et al., 2012; Pallini et al., 2017), and neurophysiological attachment research (Buchheim et al., 2017). Interest in integrating attachment theory in psychotherapy has burgeoned over the past decade. In addition to the chapters in this book, the reader is referred to other papers that describe using the AAP in different therapeutic models, such as psychodynamic and dialectical behavior therapy (e.g., Bernheim et al., 2019; Buchheim et al., 2013; George & Buchheim, 2014), and in multimodal assessment (e.g., Rorschach, Thematic Apperception Test [TAT], MMPI-2), as well as in early childhood mental health intervention programs, such as the Circle of Security (Pazzagli et al., 2014).

Training to use the AAP

Ethical use of the AAP requires training in administration and coding. Following the standard of all attachment assessments, individuals are considered reliable judges in the AAP when they have reached 80% concurrence on standard reliability sets. The first day of training delves into attachment theory and the meaning of the different attachment patterns. Subsequent days teach the coding and classification system, providing individuals with practice and reliability cases as part of the training. An alternative to reliability is for trained individuals to consult with reliable judges to code and classify their cases. Information about reliable judges available for coding is provided as part of training. In addition to the English language, training is offered in German and Italian. Training in North America uses a webinar format; training in Europe uses both in-person and webinar formats.

Conclusion

The AAP is a powerful measure of attachment for adults and adolescents. The coding dimensions define major attachment-theory concepts that are not measured in any other adult attachment assessment. It provides the field with a valid, economic, and user-friendly measure of adult attachment amenable to a range of settings and virtual administration. These elements have been shown to augment the understanding of attachment processes beyond the classification group designation and the chapters that follow demonstrate the rich contributions of the AAP to clinical practice.

Acknowledgements

AAP picture stimuli reproduced with the permission of Carol George.

References

Ainsworth, M. D. S. (1989). Attachment beyond infancy. *American Psychologist, 44*(4), 709–716. https://doi.org/doi.org/10.1037/0003-066X.44.4.709

Ainsworth, M. D. S., Blehar, M., Waters, E., & Wall, S. (1978). *Patterns of attachment: A psychological study of the Strange Situation.* Erlbaum.

Allen, J. P. (2008). The attachment system in adolescence. In J. Cassidy & P. R. Shaver (Eds.), *Handbook of attachment: Theory, research, and clinical applications* (2nd ed., pp. 419–435). Guilford Press.

Bakermans-Kranenburg, M. J., & van IJzendoorn, M. H. (2009). The first 10,000 Adult Attachment Interviews: distributions of adult attachment representations in clinical and non-clinical groups. *Attachment and Human Development, 11*(3), 223–263. https://doi.org/10.1080/14616730902814762

Bartholomew, K., & Horowitz, I. M. (1999). Attachment style among young adults: A test of a category model. *Journal of Personality and Social Psychology, 61*(2), 236–244. https://doi.org/10.1037//0022-3514.61.2.226

Bernheim, D., Gander, M., Keller, F., Becker, M., Lischke, A., Mentel, R., Freyberger, H. J., & Buchheim, A. (2019). The role of attachment characteristics in dialectical behavior therapy for patients with borderline personality disorder. *Clinical Psychology and Psychotherapy, 26*(3), 339–349. https://doi.org/10.1002/cpp.2355

Bowlby, J. (1973). *Attachment and loss: Vol. 2. Separation: Anxiety and anger.* Basic Books.

Bowlby, J. (1980). *Attachment and loss: Vol. 3. Loss: Sadness and depression.* Basic Books.

Bowlby, J. (1982). *Attachment and loss: Vol. 1. Attachment.* Basic Books. (original 1969)

Bowlby, J. (1988). *A secure base.* Basic Books.

Bretherton, I., & Munholland, K. A. (2008). Internal working models in attachment relationships. In J. Cassidy & P. R. Shaver (Eds.), *Handbook of attachment: Theory, research, and clinical applications* (2nd ed., pp. 102–127). Guilford Press.

Buchheim, A., & George, C. (2011). The representational, neurobiological and emotional foundation of attachment disorganization in borderline personality disorder and anxiety disorder. In J. Solomon & C. George (Eds.), *Disorganization of attachment and caregiving* (pp. 343–382). Guilford Press.

Buchheim, A., George, C., Guendel, H., & Viviani, M. (Eds.). (2017). *Neuroscience of human attachment*. Frontiers http://www.frontiersin.org/books/all_books; http://journal.frontiersin.org/researchtopic/3053/pdf.

Buchheim, A., Labek, K., Taubner, S., Kessler, H., Pokornoy, D., Kächele, H., Cierpka, M., Roth, G., Pogarell, O., & Karch, S. (2018). Modulation of gamma band activity and late positive potential in patients with chronic depression after psychodynamic psychotherapy. *Psychotherapy and Psychosomomatics*, *87*(4), 252–254. https://doi.org/doi: 10.1159/000488090

Buchheim, A., Labek, K., Walter, S., & Viviani, R. (2013). A clinical case study of a psychoanalytic psychotherapy monitored with functional neuroimaging. *Frontiers in Human Neuroscience*, *7*. https://doi.org/10.3389/fnhum.2013.00677

Cassidy, J., & Kobak, R. R. (1988). Avoidance and its relation to other defensive processes. In J. Belsky & T. Nezworski (Eds.), *Clinical implications of attachment* (pp. 300–323). Lawrence Erlbaum.

Cassidy, J., & Marvin, R. S., with the MacArthur Attachment Working Group. (1987–1992). *Attachment organization in preschool children: Coding guidelines*.

Crowell, J. A., Fraley, R. C., & Roisman, G. I. (2016). Measurement of individual differences in adult attachment. In J. Cassidy & P. Shaver (Eds.), *Handbook of attachment: Theory, research, and clinical applications* (3rd ed., pp. 598–638). Guilford Press.

David, R. M., Carroll, A. J., & Smith, J. D. (in press, 2021). Virtual delivery of therapeutic assessment: An empirical case study. *Journal of Personality Assessment*. Online publication. https://doi.org/10.1080/00223891.2021.1929262

George, C., Kaplan, N., & Main, M. (1984/1985/1996). *The adult attachment interview* [Doctoral dissertation, University of California]. Berkeley, CA.

George, C., & Solomon, J. (2008). The caregiving system: A behavioral systems approach to parenting. In J. Cassidy & P. R. Shaver (Eds.), *Handbook of attachment: Theory, research, and clinical applications* (2nd ed., pp. 833–856). Guilford Press.

George, C., Wargo-Aikins, J., & Lehmann, M. (2020). Using the Adult Attachment Projective Picture System (AAP) in web-based assessment: AAP web-administration *Therapeutic Assessment Connection Newletter, 8.*

George, C., & West, M. (2001). The development and preliminary validation of a new measure of adult attachment: The adult attachment projective. *Attachment and Human Development*, *3*(1), 30–61. https://doi.org/https://doi.org/10.1080/14616730010024771

George, C., & West, M. (2012). *The adult attachment projective picture system: Attachment theory and assessment in adults*. Guilford Press.

George, C., West, M., & Pettem, O. (1999). The adult attachment projective: Disorganization of adult attachment at the level of representation. In J. Solomon & C. George (Eds.), *Attachment disorganization* (pp. 462–507). Guilford Press.

Hazan, C., & Shaver, P. R. (1987). Romantic love conceptualized as an attachment process. *Journal of Personality and Social Psychology*, *52*(3), 511–524. https://doi.org/10.1037/0022-3514.52.3.511

Herrmann, A. S., Beutel, M. E., Gerzymisch, K., Lane, R. D., Pastore-Molitor, J., Wiltink, J., Zwerenz, R., Banerjee, M., & Subic-Wrana, C. (2018). The impact of attachment distress on affect-centered mentalization: An experimental study in psychosomatic patients and healthy adults. *PLoS One, 13*(4), 1–18. https://doi.org/10.1371/journal.pone.0195430

Hesse, E. (2016). The Adult Attachment Interview: Protocol, method of analysis, and selected empirical studies: 1985–2015. In J. Cassidy & P. Shaver (Eds.), *Handbook of attachment: Theory, research, and clinical applications* (3rd ed., pp. 553–597). Guilford Press.

Hesse, E., & Main, M. (2006). Frightened, threatening, and dissociative parental behavior in low-risk samples: Description, discussion, and interpretations. *Development and Psychopathology, 18*(2), 309–343. https://doi.org/10.1017/S0954579406060172

Jones-Mason, K., Allen, I. E., Hamilton, S., & Weiss, S. J. (2015). Comparative validity of the adult attachment interview and the adult attachment projective. *Attachment and Human Development, 17*(5), 429–447. https://doi.org/10.1080/14616734.2015.1075562

Liotti, G. (2004). Trauma, dissociation, and disorganized attachment: Three strands of a single braid. *Psychotherapy: Theory, Research, Practice, Training, 41*(4), 472–486. https://doi.org/10.1037/0033-3204.41.4.472

Main, M., & Cassidy, J. (1988). Categories of response to reunion with the parent at age 6: Predictable from infant attachment classifications and stable over a 1-month period. *Developmental Psychology, 24*(1), 1–12. https://doi.org/10.2307/1130394

Main, M., & Goldwyn, R. (1985–2003). *Adult attachment scoring and classification system.* [manuscript]. University of California at Berkeley.

Main, M., Goldwyn, R., & Hesse, E. (2003). *Adult Attachment scoring and classification system. Version 7.2.* Unpublished manuscript. University of California, Berkeley.

Marvin, R. S., Britner, P. A., & Russell, B. S. (2016). Normative development: The ontogeny of childhood attachment. In J. Cassidy & P. R. Shaver (Eds.), *Handbook of attachment: Theory, reserach, and clinical applications* (3rd ed., pp. 273–290). Guilford Press.

Mikulincer, M., Shaver, P. R., Cassidy, J., & Berant, E. (2009). Attachment-related defensive processes. In J. H. Obegi & E. Berant (Eds.), *Attachment theory and research in clinical work with adults* (pp. 293–327). Guilford Press.

Millon, T. (1969). *Modern psychopathology: A biosocial approach to maladaptive learning and functioning.* Saunders.

Pazzagli, C., Laghezza, L., Manaresi, F., Mazzeschi, C., & Powell, B. (2014). The circle of security parenting and parent conflict: A single case study. *Frontiers in Psychology, 5.* https://doi.org/10.3389/fpsyg.2014.00887

Slade, A. (2016). Attachment and adult psychotherapy: Theory, research, and practice. In J. Cassidy & P. Shaver (Eds.), *Handbook of attachment: Theory, research, and clinical applications* (3rd ed., pp. 759–779). Guilford Press.

Solomon, J., & George, C. (2011). Dysregulation of maternal caregiving across two generations. In J. Solomon & C. George (Eds.), *Disorganization of attachment and caregiving* (pp. 25–51). Guilford Press.

Solomon, J., George, C., & De Jong, A. (1995). Children classified as controlling at age six: Evidence of disorganized representational strategies and aggression at home and at school. *Development and Psychopathology, 7*(3), 447–463. https://doi.org/10.1017/S0954579400006623

Sroufe, L. A., Egeland, B., Carlson, E. A., & Collins, A. W. (2005). *The development of the person*. Guilford Press.

West, M., & Sheldon-Keller, A. E. (1994). *Patterns of relating: An adult attachment perspective*. Guilford Press.

Zeifman, D. M., & Hazan, C. (2016). Pair bonds as attachments: Mounting evidence in support of Bowlby's hypothesis. In J. Cassidy & P. Shaver (Eds.), *Handbook of Attachment: Theory, research, and clinical applications* (pp. 416–433). Guilford Press.

2 Implications of the AAP for psychotherapy processes and outcomes

Steffani Kizziar, Katie Kivisto, and Michael Poulakis

Many of us may have entered clinical psychology partly because of our attraction to attachment theory. Perhaps we waded into our early graduate studies believing that attachment theory was the bedrock of clinical work and theory. After all, Bowlby (1988), Ainsworth (1989), and generations of scholars demonstrated that we are profoundly relational beings and showed us how fear and the defense against it structure our personality. They taught us the conditions under which children are free to explore and when and how they are inhibited. They conveyed the essentials of attunement and sensitivity, showing how our earliest relational experiences shape the dynamic structure through which we engage with the world and in relationships.

It turns out that in most clinical psychology graduate schools, the work of understanding how attachment theory animates and informs clinical work (and potentially corrects some clinical theories and approaches) is the work of solitary study and, for a few, the subject of dissertations. Attachment theory, if mentioned at all, is typically a few bullet points on a PowerPoint about another topic. Yet, without reference to attachment, for many of us, clinical theory feels unmoored – as if relational beings can be apprehended free of the relationships that formed us – as if meaning is pried away from context. So as suggested, such questions and concerns became the stuff of dissertations.

With the help of trusted advisors, the first author crafted a project to interview clinicians who use attachment theory in their clinical work. We were specifically interested in the *Adult Attachment Projective Picture System* (AAP, George & West, 2012) as a clinical tool. Until its development, there was no sustainable method to arrive at an informed, empirically derived understanding of the attachment experience rooted in the developmental model (not romantic attachment style, e.g., Cassidy & Shaver, 2016) for the clinical arena. While some case studies published about the efficacy of the *Adult Attachment Interview* (AAI, George et al., 1984; Main et al., 1985) as a clinical tool, its form and complexity make it unsupportable for most clinical services.

There has been a significant amount of research (mostly on attachment style, not developmental pattern) that explores how attachment

DOI: 10.4324/9781003215431-3

translates into how clients approach or benefit from treatment and seek to answer the question "what works for whom?" (Fonagy et al., 1996). The results of these studies are mixed. It has further been suggested that a knowledge of attachment pattern may "diminish the risk of making interventions that, being pertinent for a given subtype, could become inefficient, or even reinforce the pathology, when applied to different ones" (Bleichmar, 1996, p. 947). So, this begs the question: Does knowing about someone's attachment pattern help the clinician apprehend the most relevant and pertinent treatment approach? Some have suggested that entering treatment informed of the client's underlying attachment strategies is ideal (e.g., Bucci et al., 2014), but none have systematically studied the impact or value of formally assessing a client's developmental attachment pattern using the AAP.

The study and rationale

The purpose of the study was to explore the impact of integrating an attachment-informed assessment using the AAP into clinical work. We were interested in the clinician's experience of understanding a client's attachment pattern and how related AAP information informs their day-to-day work with the client and if and what difference it makes to treatment experience and outcomes. The study used a qualitative design to explore the clinician's subjective experience and clinician-reported treatment outcomes. This method captures the subtleties and nuances in the clinician's experience and clinical conceptualization when informed about the client's underlying attachment pattern and the trends and common themes that emerge across practice. The data analysis process was conducted according to the principles of Consensual Qualitative Research (CQR; Hill, 2012). In the spirit of learning and discovery in which the project was undertaken, the results are conveyed in the participants' voices.[1] Their wisdom is worth sharing.

Clinician overview

The clinicians were doctoral level, primarily seasoned practitioners who practiced from various theoretical perspectives. The first provocative finding emerged from the brief demographic survey in which 40% of the clinicians identified their primary theoretical orientation as "attachment-based." Bowlby never offered specific therapeutic techniques, as one would expect from a method or orientation, although he did write about the stance and aims of an attachment-informed clinician (Bowlby, 1988). This percentage suggests that in clinical practice, attachment theory is moving from being an aspect of conceptualization to a dynamic guide for clinical practice and technique. As eloquently summarized by one participant, attachment theory has moved her position beyond participant-observer and into a co-regulator of affect through emotional attunement.

> I (understand) the therapeutic alliance through the attachment framework and understand that there's attachment activation happening in the room when I'm working with a client... So, the more I can regulate, the more sensitively I can respond, the more timely I can be, the more containing as needed versus deepening and encouraging and supporting the emotion, you know, the more I can promote metacognition and thinking. The more I can promote this kind of regulation at the brain level, I think the better secure base I'm becoming and then that promotes certain safety and that promotes their capacity to calm down and self-reflect.

Slade's (2008) contention that attachment theory "generally does not in itself suggest radically different forms of therapeutic interventions" (p. 763) needs study in light of this emerging evidence. It may be, as Slade suggests, it is not radically different interventions that make a difference but that the subtle power of the shift in perspective regarding the aims of treatment and the clinician's role in an attachment informed treatment that may be mutative.

The following sections describe the central features of clinicians' use of attachment theory and the AAP and their experiences of clients' reactions to the assessment findings.

Motivation for using the AAP

All of the clinicians agreed that the AAP was indicated for clients struggling with relational issues and clarifying trauma.

> It (AAP) has given me... a ...tool to make sense of internal relational dynamics, which I did not have... It helps me help them make sense of many of their developmental relational traumas and... their current difficulties in relationship... It helps me understand how they survived relationally.

Most clinicians talked about how the AAP helps explain to clients how their past affects their present relationships in non-pathologizing and non-shaming language, which increases a sense of self-compassion and decreases shame.

> I have found it be healing... to offer a map of their internal relational model and words for how they came to be... a relational human being today is very much rooted in how people interacted with you, how you grew up, what your understanding of relationships have

been from early on and continues to be. It helps me... de-shame some of their relational difficulties because it's... based in compassion and understanding.

I'd say the AAP... really helps people understand themselves in a much more compassionate way, in that all the behaviors they learned to protect themselves from came from these early attachments, and it's not them, it's how they learned to adapt. And the AAP more than any other test does that for me.

In terms of clarifying trauma, the AAP can be a valuable tool for those without an identified trauma history to begin to recognize the impact of chronic misattunement.

For pathological mourning and the preoccupied with personal suffering, we talk a lot about attachment trauma, and I'll use that word... because people often shame themselves for... you know, it's not like I went to war or was in a car accident or something like that... and we'll talk about how often times attachment or developmental trauma is more impactful than these one-time big T traumas.

Valuable concepts

Some clinicians found the attachment data, including the coded content and mourning classifications (see Chapter 4) provided by the AAP, such as concepts of the internalized secure base, capacity to act, synchrony, connectedness, and pathological mourning, critical to their clinical conceptualization.

I was always thinking about how trauma integrated into attachment and attachment defensive processes... I'd be looking for deactivation; I'd be looking for traumatic responses, I'd be looking for cognitive disconnection and... for anything that looked like... haven of safety or secure base... I'd be looking at the synchrony scores and (considering)... what was it about the one response, what was it about that one story, what was the context, and what could I... take away from that as a resource that I might help the client draw upon.

Attachment data and diagnosis

There was general agreement that there is no observed link between diagnosis (DSM) and attachment pattern and that diagnosis is an unhelpful, limited construct. The theme that an attachment-informed understanding promotes compassion and reduces shame was again prominent. At the same time, there was a consensus that diagnoses were a form of "labeling" and always for external purposes, for example, reimbursement, the courts, and medication.

> The DSM is just not very helpful... It's a necessary evil for reimbursement... just because somebody... meets the criteria for conduct disorder or oppositional defiant disorder... doesn't tell you much. There are multiple pathways to get to that behavior: I'm looking at the pathway.

> I use the attachment pattern as a baseline as to what's happening underneath the diagnosis... The (AAP)... elucidates the roots and causes of the narcissism, for example.

Attachment-based roles of the clinician

The participants generally agreed that the clinician's role was to provide a haven of safety and a secure base for their clients, consistent with Bowlby's (1980) view. Ainsworth (1989) viewed the haven of safety as the attachment figure providing comfort when attachment needs are activated; the secure base is the individual's capacity to explore, knowing that the attachment figure is available if exploration becomes stressful or frightening. Many agreed that establishing a haven of safety was the first step that allowed for developing a secure base, which then allowed for activation of the exploratory system and for clients to become curious about their own experience.

> (Establishing) a haven of safety is... a big piece of establishing the therapeutic relationship... the client has to feel like they can trust you... that you're on their side, that you are going to support them, and this is a place to explore painful things... Once solidified, and sometimes it takes a long time, then you can start moving into some thinking about things and conceptualizing relationships and some of the higher order cognitive skills that are associated with... internalized secure base.

Nuanced treatment approach based on attachment pattern

The majority of participants indicated that their approach to treatment varies based on the client's attachment pattern. There was general agreement that most of their practice was comprised of insecure or dysregulated individuals (i.e., incomplete pathological mourning) and that attachment patterns translated into different clinical presentations and needs. For dismissing clients, many participants identified the treatment strategy as respecting the client's defenses and gradually moving them toward integrating deactivated affect. For preoccupied clients, the treatment strategy was to focus on emotion regulation. For dysregulated clients, the treatment strategy was focused on building a sense of safety and staying present. The following provides representative descriptions of these dynamics.

> ... I know if I'm working with a dismissing person... then I don't expect we are going to get into touchy-feely topics or process anytime soon, so the defenses are to modify and that usually takes time. I want to work with them in a very pragmatic, problem-solving way, which is not usually my approach, but sometimes that's what they want... and people who are preoccupied or unresolved, well, I'm going to have to do a lot of crisis resolution and probably process its ups and downs, and it's going to be a bit of a roller coaster, but that's how they function.

> ... The failed mourners... work in their left brain a lot and so the drop down into the body into the emotional piece takes a long time and helping them understand that and really helping them sit with that like stopping them and getting in there and... just doing some of the taking deep breaths and what does your body feel like and really trying to slow them down... can help move them into the affect.

> I think about what the treatment will look like, but mainly what will be the best strategy so how do I align myself with what they need... Do they need me to help them deepen into their affect, or do they need help containing the affect? How do I regulate them? How do I stay present with them in the room based on what it is happening internally with them, because I really do think that my work with them is an attachment-based framework.

> I think we have to think very carefully about what type of treatment and how fast the treatment goes (based on attachment pattern)... The other tests suggested emotional constriction and how the client navigated the world, and the AAP gave us context as to why that was so.

Illuminating the here and now

Most participants felt that understanding the client's attachment pattern and related defense informs clinical actions in the here and now and sensitizes the clinician to the activation of defense or what is likely to trigger a defensive activation. The following provides a representative way of working with an attachment-informed treatment approach.

> ...with dismissing clients... they can fly up into their head and they can think, but once we have that classification in mind, the task... is pulling them down into their emotions but being careful and aware

that when things get too emotionally ambiguous or sticky that they're going to go back to their dismissing thinking habits and... using that to help them reflect on what they're experiencing in the room... Conversely, if you have more preoccupied individuals, then, the way you set boundaries and the way you kind of pull them out of that emotional storm looks quite different. And some of that intuitively happens clinically, but when you have the coding, you're more prepared and better able to pick up on the... defensive flavor that the client experiences.

If somebody was... unresolved for trauma... we have to handle that carefully and particularly if you look at the story that they told around it, there might be something there... so you could predict that... touching on the trauma was going to trigger this kind of response so it needed to be handled very delicately... and my thought was always how do you use whatever resources they have, so do they have capacity to act? Do they have haven of safety? Rarely in that kind of situation do you have... internalized secure base, but I'm always looking for those things... And if there's no capacity to act, and there's no haven of safety, and no ISB then you're starting at capacity to act so that's how you're going to help your client contain that trauma and then eventually... metabolize it.

The majority of respondents indicated that they did think about attachment and activation of attachment defenses in times of rupture and used this understanding to effect a repair. One participant described how they would in the past inadvertently cause ruptures with their dismissing clients because they failed to appreciate their attachment to them, which the clients could not show or articulate directly.

...I used to make this rupture with dismissing people... They come to therapy, and you feel like you're worth nothing... and then I would go on vacation with no thought that there was going to be an impact on the client... and I would be so surprised by their distress... And now I don't make that mistake... I know I'm very important to this person, but there's no way he can show it to me. And so, I'm going to act in a way that honors that. And so, I don't make the kind of ruptures I used to make because I took the Ds stance personally.

Another participant described how, while in session, they may not be explicitly or consciously thinking of the client's attachment pattern, and they saw their role as attuning to where the client is to repair empathic failures.

So with the stereotypical dismissing person, if I have an empathic failure I'm not going to move into this... sort of warm way because they would not like that... So it's more being attuned to the way they are relating to me and finding a way to make a repair that's more straightforward and direct and still have a bit of softness... to help them be able to tolerate that kind of warmth... and then with the preoccupied person, I'd want to be monitoring their anxiety and making sure I'm... kind of soothing... and then with the unresolved person I'm just... hanging on and meeting them were they are.

One participant described how he found his attachment training changed his technique and understanding from his classical psychoanalytic training.

> ...I would get... supervision around... waiting until that perfect moment to make that... affectively intense interpretation because you have to get through the defenses... I think that has its place... but thinking about things from an attachment perspective... you might only want to do that with the securely attached person or... maybe the dismissive types... who have their armor plating up and you might want to get through that. But certainly not with the preoccupied or the disorganized types, it would just be bad.

Forecasting needs for and response to treatment

The majority of the clinicians felt that one of the advantages of the AAP was that it allowed them to forecast what the client is likely going to need from treatment and the course the treatment is likely to take. As summarized by one participant, *I think that's actually one of the advantages of the AAP. It gives you insight and allows some sense of forecasting and understanding.*

One participant described how they make forecasts about how the client will respond to treatment and share that with the client. This process allows them to reference that understanding when treatment is difficult. The response is quoted in full to get an adequate understanding of the dynamics.

> ...(coder) will write Ds pathological mourning... 'fasten your seatbelts if you've got this person in therapy because if they stay in therapy and they attach to you all hell is going to break loose, and they are going to look much more symptomatic.' And I'm able, when people are in the middle of that, to explain what's going on... These Ds people will come in and say, 'this therapy is making me worse. What kind of treatment is this? I now feel worse than I did.' I'll say, 'yes, you might remember I said something to you at the beginning that something like this might happen and let me explain what is going on. Growing up you didn't have attuned attachment figures and nobody to hold your emotions, so you had to shove them down,

hold them down, and pack them away. Now, we have created an environment where you are getting all those pieces of yourself back again, and it's very, very distressing... This is not a sign of you going backwards, this is a sign of you going forward, and let's just keep working on it and I can almost bet you money if we keep doing this you're going to get to a better place. You're just in the middle of the tunnel, and you can't see the end right now.

A few participants expressed reservations about making forecasts based on attachment patterns.

I don't want to overshoot predictions because we're not good at making predictions... But that being said, I do make a general prediction about what's likely to happen in terms of treatment, which is the appeal of the attachment instrument.

There was general agreement that the AAP provided an opportunity for psychoeducation on inter- or intrapersonal dynamics. The clinicians varied in how they talked about attachment, using a range of metaphors or narrative frames, but all agreed that the AAP helped create a shared language and understanding with their clients. Again, the idea was that this attachment-informed psychoeducation promoted compassion, self-understanding, and shame reduction.

One participant offered an appropriate caution about talking to clients in terms of their specific attachment category.

My talking about attachment has changed over the years... I used to put things into categories more, and I was relying too much on this is a dismissing attachment, this is a secure attachment, and so on, and I don't do that anymore. I see it as much more on a continuum, and I see it as much more of a process of describing coping mechanisms or defensive processes... Labeling certain things strongly wasn't as compassionate and as attuned to the client...

Study limitations

The CQR methodology helps guard against bias by having multiple individual perspectives on the same data and outside auditors to protect against "group-think"; however, this study has one notable area of bias. By definition, the clinicians who use the AAP in their practice believe in the efficacy of assessing and understanding a client's attachment pattern. They enthusiastically embraced the AAP to that end. The researchers tried to counterbalance that bias by carefully understanding the specific implications and impact of attachment understanding on clinical work. The interviews emphasized actual experiences with clients with known and understood attachment patterns, not theoretical beliefs. And while the qualitative method as described by CQR is rich and nuanced, what emerges remains a single vantage point on the research questions formulated to guide the study. Ideally, one would use mixed methods and include a quantitative portion about client outcomes alongside the more subjective, qualitative data. In hindsight, of course, some questions should have been included, such as "what is the difference in treatment when you know a client's attachment pattern versus those when you go in 'blind?'"

Conclusions

This research took us into the clinical rooms and minds of those clinicians who use the AAP to inform and enrich their clinical work. They provided an intriguing and exciting glimpse into the possibilities of such work and a beautiful rendering of what happens when theory meets practice. The notion that "attachment" is becoming an orientation in itself is a particularly intriguing finding – along with the specific interventions and therapeutic approach that flow from this stance.

This work suggests that an attachment-informed perspective lends itself to empathic understanding of the client's fears and needs as they are awakened in the therapeutic relationship and how that understanding illuminates transferential issues, strengthens the therapeutic alliance, and guides therapeutic intervention. Using an attachment lens, these clinicians understand the psychological survival function of defenses as protecting the client from intolerable experiences and affect (George & West, 2012; Holmes, 2001; Slade, 2008). Such an understanding leads to a reformulation of the client's defenses from treatment resistance to a fight for survival, as the function of defenses is for the protection of self and others. In this, maladaptive responses are understood as necessary survival mechanisms that make sense given the client's history. It appropriately locates the "wrong" in the client's story. It has the effect of shifting the therapeutic task from "digging for unacknowledged truth" (Slade, 2008, p. 776) to functioning as a secure base, with all the elements of responsive attunement implied therein (Farber et al., 1995).

These voices made it clear that many clinicians adjust their interpersonal stance and technique in response to different attachment patterns. It appears these clinicians flexibly respond in and out of style depending on the demands of the clinical moment, all the while holding firmly in mind the underlying relational dynamics (i.e., attachment pattern) in play. From this informed perspective, they navigate rupture and repairs, which helps solidify their role as a secure base and affords the client a new relational experience.

An important recurrent theme that emerged was the strength of the AAP. It provides a non-pathologizing way of explaining the client's difficulties, not simply a description of symptoms but a diagnosis. Instead, it describes the factors that worked together to create the presenting constellation of symptoms. It moves the discussion beyond what is wrong with the client to provide a new narrative of what happened to them and how they had to adapt to their (often) less than optimal childhood environment. Repeatedly, clinicians reported this had the effect of reducing shame and offering the client a new, more compassionate narrative of their lives.

As Main and colleagues (1985) demonstrated with the AAI, narrative competence and the capacity to reflect on one's own story is the hallmark of attachment security. Intriguingly, insecure individuals can use their familiarity with the results of the AAP to begin to reflect on their life stories from different, more coherent perspectives. As Holmes (2001) describes, "Ultimately, emotional security comes from the experience of being understood" (p. 42); directly engaging the results of the AAP offers clients a profound understanding of themselves in conversation with a (potential) attachment figure at the outset of treatment.

There was widespread agreement that the clinician's role is to function as a secure base once they have established a haven of safety. Clients then had the freedom to begin to explore their inner world and bear the anguish of facing and integrating what had previously been split off, disavowed, or unnamed. This exploration has clear implications for technique as clinicians initiate treatment with their insecure clients. A haven of safety is built through availability and consistency, while a secure base is built through attunement and affect regulation. It appears the former has to be strong enough for the client to bear the latter.

These clinicians affirmed that they are more likely to "use language and metaphors that will be meaningful, evocative, and experience-near for the client" (Slade, 2008, p. 774) when they better understand and appreciate the needs, fears, and longing underlying the client's internal working model. It seems likely that a therapeutic relationship that is "experience-near" has a better chance of helping clients with "knowing what [they] are not supposed to know and feeling what [they] are not supposed to feel" (Bowlby, 1988, p. 99).

The introduction of the AAP has expanded the ability to track the nuances of attachment experience as described by Bowlby. The AAP has moved the field from simple categorical designations to a more sophisticated and nuanced expression of the individual's attachment experience and its consequences. This research is just the beginning of this conversation. The hope is that this will inspire future research that subjects all the findings to further analysis and empirical testing.

Note

1 Participants are quoted directly and presented in italics. They were redacted only for brevity and clarity, and the redactions are noted.

References

Ainsworth, M. D. S. (1989). Attachment beyond infancy. *American Psychologist, 44*(4), 709–716. https://doi.org/10.1037/0003-066X.44.4.709

Bleichmar, H. (1996). Some subtypes of depression and their implications for psychoanalytic treatment. *International Journal of Psychoanalysis, 77*(5), 935–961. PPMID: 8933219.

Bowlby, J. (1988). *A secure base: Parent-child attachment and healthy human development.* Basic Books.

Bucci, S., Roberts, N., Danquah, A., & Berry, K. (2014). Using attachment theory to inform the design and delivery of mental health services: A systemic review of the literature. *Psychology and Psychotherapy: Theory, Research, and Practice, 88*(1), 1–20. https://doi.org/10.1111.papt.12029.

Cassidy, J., & Shaver, P. R. (2016). *Handbook of attachment: Theory, research, and clinical applications.* Guilford Press.

Farber, B., Lippert, R., & Nevas, D. (1995). The therapist as attachment figure. *Psychotherapy, 32*(2), 204–212. https://doi.org/10.1037/0033-3204.32.2.204.

Fonagy, P., Leigh, T., Steele, M., Steele, H., Kennedy, R., Mattoon, G., Target, M., & Gerber, A. (1996). The relation of attachment status, psychiatric classification, and response to psychotherapy. *Journal of Consulting and Clinical Psychology, 64*(4), 22–31. https://doi.org/10.1037//0022–006x.641.22.

George, C., Kaplan, N., & Main, M. (1984/1985/1996). *The Adult Attachment Interview* [Doctoral dissertation, University of California]. Berkeley, CA.

George, C., & West, M. (2012). *The adult attachment projective picture system: Attachment theory and assessment in adults.* Guilford Press.

Hill, C. (2012). *Consensual qualitative research: A practical resource for investigating social science phenomena.* American Psychological Association.

Holmes, J. (2001). *The search for the secure base: Attachment theory and psychotherapy.* Routledge.

Main, M., Kaplan, N., & Cassidy, Y. (1985). Security in infancy, childhood and adulthood: A move to the level of representation. In I. Bretherton & E. Waters (Eds.), *Growing points of attachment: Theory and research. Monographs of the society for research in child development, 50* (1–2, Serial No. 209, pp. 60–106). https://doi.org/10.2307/3333827

Slade, A. (2008). The implications of attachment theory and research for adult psychotherapy: Research and Clinical Perspectives. In J. Cassidy & Shaver, P. (Eds.) *Handbook of attachment: Theory, research, and clinical applications* (2nd ed., pp. 762–782). Guilford Press.

3 Clinical and neurobiological applications of the AAP in adults and adolescents
Therapeutic implications

Anna Buchheim and Manuela Gander

This chapter summarizes the role of the Adult Attachment Projective Picture System (AAP) in our work examining the neurobiological underpinnings of emotion regulation, psychopathology, and psychotherapy in adults and adolescents. Adolescence is a period of profound transformation in which individuals develop an integrated sense of self and autonomy from parents (Allen & Tan, 2016). Our research has particular clinical relevance. Even though attachment conceptualizations of adolescence provide a helpful framework for understanding developmental processes and transitions, there is a paucity of attachment research and its clinical implications for adolescents (Allen & Tan, 2016; Gander et al., 2016). The chapter begins with our studies on the neuroscience of emotion regulation describing our unique AAP methodology and the results of these neuroimaging and endocrinological studies. We then examine unresolved attachment in psychopathology and psychotherapy research, largely neglected areas of study in these domains. In this respect, examining the unresolved attachment representation and attachment-related material might help advance disorder-specific characteristics of mental disorders in different clinical samples.

The neural correlates of attachment: Using the AAP in neurophysiological studies

Research on the neuroscience of human attachment represents a broad spectrum of contemporary approaches to investigating biologically based systems that guide the cognitive and emotional processes of intimate and significant relationships. This spectrum includes studies and theoretical reviews that discuss neurobiological substrates (fMRI, EEG, psychophysiology, endocrine parameters, genetic polymorphisms) using a range of psychometric approaches to attachment assessment (interview, e.g., Adult Attachment Interview, AAI, George et al., 1984), the AAP (George & West, 2012), and self-report questionnaire (e.g., Relationship Scales Questionnaire, Griffin & Bartholomew, 1994). In sum, this growing body of research has broadened our understanding of how

DOI: 10.4324/9781003215431-4

attachment is related to impaired emotion regulation (for an overview, see Buchheim, Hörz-Sagstetter et al., 2017).

We have used the AAP in neurobiological attachment research, including fMRI studies measuring the neural correlates of human attachment in adults and adolescents (Buchheim, Erk et al. 2006; Buchheim, George et al. 2006; Bernheim et al., 2022; Buchheim et al., 2008, 2012, 2018; Gander et al., 2022). Our first neuroimaging study was a methodological test of the feasibility of using the AAP in a neuroimaging setting (Buchheim, Erk et al., 2006). In this community sample, participants told AAP stories while presenting the picture stimuli in the scanner. The results showed that the AAP can successfully be administered in an fMRI environment and that the participants' narratives could be coded using the standardized AAP classification system. The most exciting finding of our initial work was that Unresolved participants showed significantly more activation of limbic areas when administering the AAP. This results pattern in the actual brain scans showed the challenges to emotion regulation faced by Unresolved participants.

Based on these results, we continued this line of research to investigate the neural correlates of attachment trauma in patients with Borderline Personality Disorder (BPD) compared to healthy controls (Buchheim et al., 2018). We found that Unresolved attachment in both groups demonstrated enhanced amygdala activation, but activation in the controls appeared to be balanced by frontal activations and top-down control. This finding pointed to a possible neural mechanism in BPD patients with Unresolved attachment trauma (the attachment pattern most associated with BPD in the literature) that explained their inability to regulate attachment distress.

Using the same sample, we also explored (Buchheim et al., 2008) the neurophysiological correlates of trauma using the language-based trauma indicators in the AAP narratives (segregated systems, see Chapter 4) that participants produced when they were telling stories in the fMRI scanner. The AAP approach to trauma differentiates "normative" segregated systems pulled for by a picture from unusual or frightening indicators. We, therefore, compared the normative segregated systems language and narratives with those indicating trauma. Being confronted with the alone pictures was difficult, especially for the BPD patients, triggering more traumatic dysregulation in the narratives than observed in the stories of the dyadic AAP picture scenes. The alone picture response patterns showed higher activations in brain regions associated with pain and fear (dorsal anterior cingulate cortex) than healthy controls. These findings provided the first objective evidence of possible mechanisms related to dysregulated affect associated with the "fearful intolerance of aloneness" proposed as characteristic of individuals with BPD (Gunderson, 1996).

Years later, Bernheim et al. (2022) replicated these findings in an fMRI study using an adapted AAP paradigm developed by Buchheim et al. (2012). What was unique about this paradigm was eliminating the need for participants to speak in the scanner by showing the AAP pictures with written statements from the participants' AAPs completed prior to the scanner portion of the study. We developed a comparison control set of pictures that portrayed neutral descriptive statements. For example, a personalized statement extracted from the AAP Window story was "A girl is incarcerated in that big room." A neutral statement example for the same stimulus was "There is a window with curtains on the left and on the right." Trials alternated between the personally relevant and neutral in seven AAP picture stimuli groups. As in our original 2008 study, BPD patients showed emotion regulation problem challenges with increased fMRI-activation in brain areas associated with fear and pain compared to healthy controls when the visual stimuli were their personalized AAPs.

In addition to our basic research, we integrated neuroimaging into our psychotherapy research to study the effects and mechanisms of psychotherapy. While most studies have investigated short-time therapies, Buchheim et al. (2012) conducted the first fMRI study examining long-term psychodynamic treatments on chronically depressed patients using the fMRI personalized AAP paradigm (see Chapter 10 for a single case). The effects were localized in brain emotion regulation areas, including the left amygdala extending laterally into the anterior hippocampus and toward the middle temporal gyrus.

Buchheim et al. (2018, 2019) also used this personalized AAP fMRI paradigm in an EEG setting with the same sample of depressed patients. The findings demonstrated significant modulations of gamma-band activity and late positive potential after psychodynamic psychotherapy, indicating a psychotherapy effect. This neurophysiological evidence demonstrated improved emotion regulation one year after treatment. Additionally, we demonstrated high convergent validity between the AAI and the AAP in $N = 30$ participants, $\kappa = 0.89$ (ASE = 0.112), $p < 0.001$, simple agreement 94%, and significant change of attachment after treatment in both measures (Buchheim et al., 2018).

Neurophysiological and endocrinological regulatory studies using the AAP

Results from infant and adult studies suggest that a secure attachment is an essential buffer for the physiological reactivity to attachment-related stressors. The buffer effect is because secure individuals balance attachment and exploration, flexibly using their attachment figures as a haven of safety and secure base and expressing their emotions directly and openly. Regulatory buffering is evidenced on a physiological level by lower adrenocortical activity and lower increases in heart rate and skin conductance levels when secure individuals experience stressful attachment-related situations. On the other hand, attachment insecurity creates deficits in emotion regulation. These deficits manifest in insecure-preoccupied individuals as expressed anger and less autonomy than secures. Deficits manifest in insecure-dismissing individuals compared with secures are dismissal and deactivation of attachment distress and independence. Under stress, individuals in these insecure groups demonstrate heightened physiological reactivity (Gander & Buchheim, 2015).

Our research group has shown that the AAP can be used as an attachment-related stimulus to examine neurobiological regulatory pathways, including the oxytocinergic system in clinical and community samples of adults and adolescents (Buchheim et al., 2016; Fuchshuber et al., 2020). In one of our first psychosomatics studies, we investigated cardiovascular responses during the AAP procedure in adult patients with hypertension (Balint et al., 2016). The patients showed a significant increase in blood pressure, heart rate, and rate pressure product in response to the AAP, providing a physiological window into how the AAP activates physiological regulation of the attachment system (Balint et al., 2016).

The study of neurophysiological correlates of attachment in adolescents is a relatively untapped area of research. In the only adolescent study to date, Gander and Buchheim (2015) used the AAP to examine neurophysiological parameters during the AAP administration. The study results failed to confirm the patterns of physiological functioning reported in studies of infants and adults (Beijersbergen et al., 2008). This contradictory finding raises an important question of differences in reactivity to stressors during adolescence. In a subsequent study, our study group used the AAP with adolescents to measure autonomic imbalance during attachment-related stressful situations using heart-rate variability (Bryant & Hutanamon, 2018), a central index of physiological emotion regulation. The significant finding of this study was that secure adolescents showed more flexible heart rate variability from baseline when responding to the AAP compared to insecure adolescents. As a further validation, we found high convergent correspondence with the AAI (94%, $\kappa = 0.89$, $p < 0.001$, for the two-group classifications (resolved-Unresolved) and 81%, $\kappa = 0.81$, $p < 0.001$, for the four-group classifications) (Gander et al., 2022). The regulatory flexibility of secure adolescents suggests these adolescents had developed healthy ways of dealing with attachment-related distress when attachment is activated. These results add to a body of research showing that attachment security fosters the development of adaptive ways of coping with negative emotions (Allen & Miga, 2010).

Adult and adolescent Unresolved attachment: Using the AAP in psychopathology and psychotherapy research

A large body of studies in different psychiatric groups demonstrate associations between attachment patterns, symptom severity, and treatment outcome (e.g., Maxwell et al., 2017). The Unresolved attachment pattern is a significant predictor of social and cognitive difficulties and psychopathology (Bakermans-Kranenburg & van IJzendoorn et al., 2009). Neurobiological research provides additional support for links between the Unresolved pattern and symptom severity in psychiatric adult patients like BPD (Buchheim et al., 2017; Buchheim & Diamond, 2018).

Our research group was interested in using the AAP in adult clinical samples to explore the physiological and neurobiological regulatory differences associated with Unresolved attachment. Jobst et al. (2016) examined the differences between organized (Secure, Dismissing, Preoccupied) and Unresolved BPD patients during a Cyberball experiment. The Cyberball experiment is a well-established social exclusion paradigm that activates social pain in humans. We found evidence for emotional regulation difficulties in patients with Unresolved than organized attachment. Unresolved patients demonstrated lower oxytocin plasma levels at every time point during the experiment. We interpreted this differential pattern to suggest that oxytocin release after the experience of social exclusion reflects a neuroendocrine reaction to broken relationships. The lower oxytocin levels in Unresolved borderline patients may reflect their impaired ability to repair broken relationships and induce a prosocial orientation (King-Casas et al., 2008). Bauriedl-Schmidt et al. (2017) conducted a similar study with depressive adult patients.

Our research group was also inspired by the growing literature addressing attachment in adolescent patients. We focused on anorexia nervosa and major depression: the two most common disorders encountered in adolescent psychiatric settings. Numerous studies focusing on attachment issues and family dynamics in eating disorders have been published in the last decades (see for review Gander et al., 2016). The most recent narrative-based research reported a predominance of the Unresolved pattern in adults with anorexia nervosa (Delvecchio et al., 2014). However, we know little about anorexic adolescents with Unresolved attachment.

Gander, Sevecke et al. (2018) evaluated the specific forms of traumatic dysregulation in the AAP stories of adolescents with anorexia nervosa compared with teens with a major depressive episode to investigate for the first time in the literature the potential differences between these groups. Our results showed that anorexic adolescents showed more isolation and dissolution of boundaries between life and death (i.e., spectral) in their AAP stories portraying the projected self as alone.

The following narrative illustrates these themes in a 15-year-old girl with the restrictive type of anorexia nervosa. Her isolation is prominent in the story to Bench[1]:

There is a young girl. She is sitting on a bench in her school. She wants to ***curl up into a little ball. She just wants to disappear from this world.*** Maybe she was ***teased*** by her schoolmates. ***And she has nobody who can help her because she is completely alone.*** She feels alone and ***isolated.*** And she thinks there is ***no way out of this situation.*** She is crying and ***doesn't know what to do.*** I don't think there is a happy ending. The other kids are going to ***tease*** her again and again. ***And she won't get any help, not even from her parents,*** because her problems are not important to them.	Traumatic derealization Traumatic shame Trauma Trauma Disconnect Disconnect, Trauma

The main character (projected self) experiences overwhelming feelings of isolation and shame in this story. Adaptive disconnection defenses fail to divert attention from the self's distress, and the girl in the story remains dysregulated. Attachment figures are inaccessible and fail to protect her. Consequently, the girl feels abandoned and wants to disappear because she cannot contain these threatening feelings.

Gander, Sevecke et al. (2018) found that anorexic patients had a considerable amount of trauma-specific material in their stories. They also reported moderate to severe levels of traumatic childhood experiences on the Childhood Trauma Questionnaire; however, they tended to minimize these experiences when asked to designate on the questionnaire how distressing they were. By comparison, adolescents with a major depressive episode reported more intense levels of childhood trauma. Further, they did not attempt to minimize their situation. Their AAPs showed self-representations depicting a chronic state of feeling endangered without attachment figure protection. This AAP approach used in this study added a deeper understanding of the representational nuances of childhood attachment trauma for these adolescents than available in the literature to date. Based on these findings, we developed a model that visualizes how experiences of child abuse and neglect might be related to disorder-specific attachment themes that lead to a dysregulation of the attachment system in these adolescent patients.

Gander et al. (2020) expanded this model to examine the mechanisms by which Unresolved attachment partly explains how childhood maltreatment impacts adolescent development and psychopathology. We found that Unresolved attachment mediated the relationship between childhood maltreatment and personality functioning. In particular, the associations between emotional abuse and the developmental domains of identity, empathy, self-direction, and intimacy were mediated by the sheer amount of Unresolved AAP narrative material. We used the amount of material to represent traumatic intensity. The results suggest that adolescents with higher-intensity Unresolved attachment have lowered resilience to childhood experiences resulting in more severe personality problems.

Gander et al. (2021) extended this in-depth AAP trauma analysis approach to an inpatient sample of adolescents with non-suicidal self-injury disorder. Our results revealed severe levels of representational trauma material in these patients, particularly representations of the self as helpless and endangered without protection during interpersonal conflicts. These self-representations left them in a chronic state of attachment dysregulation.

The results of these studies have important clinical implications for attachment-based treatments. Including these results in interventions that focus on parent-teen relationships and dyadic affect, regulation might allow these teens to develop more adaptive emotion regulation strategies and effective interpersonal relationships. Intervention strategies helping them face the nuances of their Unresolved attachment might lead to more adaptive emotion regulation strategies, particularly in interpersonal relationships. This approach might benefit adolescent patients with severe mental disorders who often need costly prolonged hospitalization.

Most recently, Lenhart et al.'s (2022) study of anorexic Unresolved adolescent patients showed how their representational status was apparent in the gray matter plasticity of brain structures after treatments involved in emotion regulation, processing of inner mental processes, fear of gaining weight, and body dissatisfaction. We found less region-specific grey matter increases in the anorexic patients associated with attachment trauma, which might indicate persistent emotion regulation deficits after traditional psychotherapeutic and nutritional treatment.

We agree with Kobak and Kerig's (2015) suggestion that adolescent patients might particularly benefit from attachment-based treatments, and our studies show the importance of targeting specific AAP-generated content and defenses. We used this approach with adolescent patients to help plan therapeutic interventions (Gander, Diamond et al., 2018; Gander & Sevecke, 2015; Gander et al., 2017). In this regard, the AAP has also been a viable tool to uncover attachment-related underlying symptom causes, formulate therapeutic goals, and develop a treatment plan in patients with severe traumatization (see also George & Buchheim, 2014).

More broadly, can we move patients, especially Unresolved patients, toward security? This question has been at the forefront for some clinical attachment researchers who postulated that attachment-based treatments for adolescents (Kobak & Kerig, 2015) and adults (Slade, 2008) could potentially increase attachment security and reduce psychopathological symptoms. In this context, assessing changes in an individual's attachment patterns and evaluating the dynamic process of change in attachment relationships might be an exciting approach in testing the effectiveness of specific interventions for psychiatric disorders characterized by severe impairments in interpersonal relationships. Studies in the field of psychodynamic psychotherapy have demonstrated a change in attachment patterns for patients with BPDs during Transference-Focused Psychotherapy (Buchheim et al., 2017; Levy et al., 2006) and depression (Buchheim et al., 2012, 2018, 2019). Moreover, studies demonstrated significant changes in attachment features towards attachment security and an improved ability to emotionally integrate autobiographical attachment-related material after one year of Dialectic Behavioral Therapy (Bernheim et al., 2017, 2019). Evaluating changes in attachment representations throughout treatment or evaluating sustained changes at the end of treatment is facilitated by the user-friendly economical design of the AAP (see Finn, Chapter 8, in this volume).

Conclusions

The AAP provided a unique approach for our research group to examine regulatory processes and the clinical implications of attachment for adults and adolescents. Many of our studies focused on the Unresolved attachment classification, which has been neglected in our domains of study and is especially relevant to clinical practice. The AAP served as a powerful paradigm for investigating neurobiological and neurophysiological correlates of attachment and regulation. Moreover, we showed that the AAP is valid for evaluating changes in attachment-related issues during the course and after psychotherapeutic treatment. Our work suggests that clinicians would benefit from looking more deeply into attachment patterns than the attachment group. Paying close attention to how the AAP coding dimensions may guide treatment and understanding symptom reduction in adult and adolescent groups. This focus could also be essential for subsequent studies and interventions related to the cost-effectiveness of attachment-based treatments compared to other evidence-based psychotherapies, particularly for younger patients.

Note

1 Italics = defenses; bold = trauma

References

Allen, J. P., & Miga, E. M. (2010). Attachment in adolescence: A move to the level of emotion regulation. *Journal of Social and Personal Relationships, 27*(2), 181–190. https://doi.org/10.1177/0265407509360898

Allen, J. P., & Tan, S. T. (2016). The multiple facets of attachment in adolescence. In J. Cassidy & P. R. Shaver (Eds.), *Handbook of attachment: Theory, research, and clinical applications* (3rd ed., pp. 399–415). Guilford Press.

Ammaniti, M., van IJzendoorn, M. H., Speranza, A. M., & Tambelli, R. (2000). Internal working models of attachment during late childhood and early adolescence: An exploration of stability and change. *Attachment and Human Development, 2*(3), 328–346. https://doi.org/10.1080/14616730010001587

Bakermans-Kranenburg, M. J., & van IJzendoorn, M. H. (2009). The first 10,000 Adult Attachment Interviews: Distributions of adult attachment representations in clinical and non-clinical groups. *Attachment and Human Development, 11*(3), 223–263. https://doi.org/10.1080/14616730902814762.

Balint, E. M., Gander, M., Pokorny, D., Funk, A., Waller, C., & Buchheim, A. (2016). High prevalence of insecure attachment in patients with primary hypertension. *Frontiers in Psychology, 7*, 1087. https://doi.org/10.3389/fpsyg.2016.01087

Bauriedl-Schmidt, C., Jobst, A., Gander, M., Seidl, E., Sabaß, L., Sarubin, N., Mauer, S., Padberg, F., & Buchheim, A. (2017). Attachment representations, patterns of emotion regulation, and social exclusion in patients with chronic and episodic depression and healthy controls. *Journal of Affective Disorders, 210*, 130–138. https://doi.org/10.1016/j.jad.2016.12.030

Beijersbergen, M. D., Bakermans-Kranenburg, M. J., van Ijzendoorn, M. H., & Juffer, F. (2008). Stress regulation in adolescents: Physiological reactivity during the adult attachment interview and conflict interaction. *Child Development, 79*(6), 1707–1720. https://doi.org/10.1111/j.1467-8624.2008.01220.x

Bernheim, D., Becker, M., Gander, M., Lischke, A., Mentel, R., Buchheim, A., & Freyberger, H. J. (2017). Influence and change of self-directedness in dialectical behavior therapy. *Psychiatrische Praxis, 44*(5), 266–273. https://doi.org/10.1055/s-0042-104096

Bernheim, D., Buchheim, A., Domin, M., Mentel, R., & Lotze, M. (2022): Neural correlates of attachment representation in patients with borderline personality disorder using a personalized fMRI task. *Frontiers in Human Neuroscience.* https://www.frontiersin.org/articles/10.3389/fnhum.2022.810417/abstract

Bernheim, D., Gander, M., Keller, F., Becker, M., Lischke, A., Mentel, R., Freyberger, H. J., & Buchheim, A. (2019). The role of attachment characteristics in dialectical behavior therapy for patients with borderline personality disorder. *Clinical Psychology and Psychotherapy, 26*(3), 339–349. https://doi.org/10.1002/cpp.2355

Bryant, R. A., & Hutanamon, T. (2018). Activating attachments enhances heart rate variability. *PLoS One, 13,* e0151747. https://doi.org/10.1371/journal.pone.0151747

Buchheim, A., & Diamond, D. (2018). Attachment and borderline personality disorder. *Psychiatric Clinics of North America, 41*(4), 651–668. https://doi.org/10.1016/j.psc.2018.07.010.

Buchheim, A., Erk, S., George, C., Kächele, H., Ruchsow, M., Spitzer, M., Kircher, T., & Walter, H. (2006). Measuring attachment representation in an fMRI environment: A pilot study. *Psychopathology, 39*(3), 144–152. https://doi.org/10.1159/000091800

Buchheim, A., Erk, S., George, C., Kächele, H., Kircher, T., Martius, P., Pokorny, D., Ruchsow, M., Spitzer, M., & Walter, H. (2008). Neural correlates of attachment trauma in borderline personality disorder: A functional magnetic resonance imaging study. *Psychiatry Research, 163*(3), 223–235. https://doi.org/10.1016/j.pscychresns.2007.07.001

Buchheim, A., Erk, S., George, C., Kächele, H., Martius, P., Pokorny, D., Spitzer, M., & Walter, H. (2016). Neural response during the activation of the attachment system in patients with borderline personality disorder: An fMRI study. *Frontiers in Human Neuroscience, 10,* 389. [Online 2 August 2016. https://doi.org/10.3389/fnhum.2016.00389]

Buchheim, A., & George, C. (2011). Attachment disorganization in borderline personality disorder and anxiety disorder. In J. Solomon & C. George (Eds.), *Disorganized attachment and caregiving* (pp. 343–383). Guilford Press.

Buchheim, A., George, C., Erk, S., Kächele, H., & Walter, H. (2006). Measuring attachment representation in an fMRI environment: Concepts and assessment. *Psychopathology, 39*(3), 144–152. https://doi.org/10.1159/000091800

Buchheim, A., George, C., Gündel, H., & Viviani, R. (2017). Editorial: Neuroscience of human attachment. *Frontiers in Human Neuroscience, 11,* 36. [Online published 24 March 2017]. https://doi.org/10.3389/fnhum.2017.00136

Buchheim, A., Hörz-Sagstetter, S., Döring, S., Rentrop, M., Schuster, P., Buchheim, P., Pokorny, D., & Fischer-Kern, M. (2017). Change of unresolved attachment in borderline personality disorder: RCT study of transference-focused psychotherapy. *Psychotherapy and Psychosomatics, 86*(5), 314–316. [Online: https://doi.org/10.1159/000460257]. https//:doi.org/10.3389/fpsyg.2018.00173

Buchheim, A., Labek, K., Taubner, S., Kessler, H., Pokorny, D., Kächele, H., Cierpka, M., Roth, G., Pogarell, O., & Karch, S. (2018). Modulation of gamma band activity and late positive potential in patients with chronic depression after psychodynamic psychotherapy. *Psychotherapy and Psychosomatics, 87*(4), 252–254. https://doi.org/ 10.1159/000488090. PMID:29768272

Buchheim, A., Viviani, R., Kessler, H., Kächele, H., Cierpka, M., Roth, G., George, C., Kernberg, O. F., Bruns, G., & Taubner, S. (2012). Changes in prefrontal-limbic function in major depression after 15 months of long-term psychotherapy. *PLoS One, 7*(3), e33745. https://doi.org/10.1371/journal.pone.0033745

Buchheim, A., Viviani, R., Kessler, H., Tabner, S., Kächele, H., Roth, G., Pogarell, O., Karch, S., & Labek, K. (2019). Neurophysiological changes in depressed patients with unresolved attachment during long-term psychotherapy. *Psychotherapy and Psychosomatics, 88*(suppl 1), 19. [Online: https://www.karger.com/Article/Pdf/502467]. https://doi.org/10.1159/000502467

Delvecchio, E., Di Riso, D., Salcuni, S., Lis, A., & George, C. (2014). Anorexia and attachment: Dysregulated defense and pathological mourning. *Frontiers in Psychology, 5*, 1218. https://doi.org/10.3389/fpsyg.2014.01218

Fuchshuber, J., Tatzer, J., Hiebler-Ragger, M., Trinkl, F., Kimmerle, A., Rinner, A., Buchheim, A., Schrom, S., Rinner, B., Leber, K., Pieber, T., Weiss, E., Lewis, A. J., Kapfhammer, H. P., & Unterrainer, H. F. (2020). The influence of an attachment-related stimulus on oxytocin reactivity in poly-drug users undergoing maintenance therapy compared to healthy controls. *Frontiers in Psychiatry, 11*. https://doi.org/10.3389/fpsyt.2020.460506

Gander, M., & Buchheim, A. (2015). Attachment classification, psychophysiology and frontal EEG asymmetry across the lifespan: A review. *Frontiers in Human Neuroscience, 9*, 79. https://doi.org/10.3389/fnhum.2015.00079

Gander, M., Buchheim, A., Bock, A., Steppan, M., Sevecke, K., & Goth, K. (2020). Unresolved attachment mediates the relationship between childhood trauma and maladaptive personality functioning in adolescence. *Journal of Personality Disorders, 34*(Issue supplement B), 84–103. https://doi.org/10.1521/pedi_2020_34_468

Gander, M., Diamond, D., Buchheim, A., & Sevecke, K. (2018). Use of the adult attachment projective picture system in the formulation of a case of an adolescent refugee with PTSD. *Journal of Trauma and Dissociation, 19*(5), 1–24. https://doi.org/10.1080/15299732.2018.1451803

Gander, M., Fuchs, M., Jahnke-Majorkovits, A.-C., Buchheim, A., Bock, A., & Sevecke, K. (2021). Non-suicidal self-injury and attachment trauma in adolescent inpatients with psychiatric disorders. *Comprehensive Psychiatry, 111*, 152273. http://doi.org/10.1016/j.comppsych.2021.152273

Gander, M., George, C., Pokorny, D., & Buchheim, A. (2016). Assessing attachment representations in adolescents: Discriminant validation of the adult attachment projective picture system. *Child Psychiatry and Human Development, 48*, 270–282. https://doi.org/10.1007/s10578-016-0639-2

Gander, M., Karabatsiakis, A., Nuderscher, K., & Buchheim, A. (2022). Secure attachment representations buffer physiological reactivity in response to attachment-related stressors. *Frontiers in Human Neuroscience [Epub ahead of print].* https://doi.org/10.3389/inhum2022.806987

Gander, M., Oberhofer, B., & Sevecke, K. (2017). Integration of attachment-related aspects into art therapy in adolescent personality disorders. *Persönlichkeitsstörungen: Theorie und Therapie, 19*(3), 213–223.

Gander, M., & Sevecke, K. (2015). Attachment issues in an adolescent girl with a borderline personality disorder. *Persönlichkeitsstörungen: Theorie und Therapie, 19*(3), 213–223.

Gander, M., Sevecke, K., & Buchheim, A. (2015). Eating disorders in adolescence: Attachment issues from a developmental perspective. *Frontiers in Psychology, 6*, 1136. https://doi.org/10.3389/fpsyg.2015.01136

Gander, M., Sevecke, K., & Buchheim, A. (2018). Disorder-specific attachment characteristics and experiences of childhood abuse and neglect in adolescents with anorexia nervosa and a major depressive episode. *Clinical Psychology and Psychotherapy, 25*(6), 894–906. https://doi.org/10.1002/cpp.2324

George, C., & Buchheim, A. (2014). Use of the adult attachment projective picture system in psychodynamic psychotherapy with a severely traumatized patient. *Frontiers in Psychology, 5.* https://doi.org/10.3389/fpsyg.2014.00865

George, C., Kaplan, N., & Main, M. (1984). *The Adult Attachment Interview* [Unpublished interview, University of California]. Berkeley, CA. Initially published in C. George's dissertation.

George, C., & West, M. L. (2012). *The adult attachment projective picture system: Attachment theory and assessment in adults.* Guilford Press.

Griffin, D. W., & Bartholomew, K. (1994). Models of the self and other: Fundamental dimensions underlying measures of adult attachment. *Journal of Personality and Social Psychology, 67*(3), 430–445. https://doi.org/10.1037/0022-3514.67.3.430

Gunderson, J. G. (1996). The borderline patient's intolerance of aloneness: Insecure attachments and therapist availability. *American Journal of Psychiatry, 153*(6), 752–758. https://doi.org/10.1176/ajp.153.6.752

Jobst, A., Padberg, F., Mauer, M. C., Daltrozzo, T., Bauriedl-Schmidt, C., Sabass, L., Sarubin, N., Falkai, P., Rennberg, B., Zill, P., Gander, M., & Buchheim, A. (2016). Lower oxytocin plasma levels in borderline patients with unresolved attachment representations. *Frontiers in Human Neuroscience, 10*, 125. https://doi.org/10.3389/fnhum.2016.00125

Joubert, D., Webster, L., & Hackett, R. K. (2012). Unresolved attachment status and trauma-related symptomatology in maltreated adolescents: An examination of cognitive mediators. *Child Psychiatry and Human Development, 43*(3), 471–483. https://doi.org/10.1007/s10578-011-0276-8

Kerns, K. A. (2008). Attachment in middle childhood. In J. Cassidy & P. R. Shaver (Eds.), *Handbook of attachment: Theory, research, and clinical applications* (2nd ed., pp. 366–382). Guilford Press.

King-Casas, B., Sharp, C., Lomax-Bream, L., Lohrenz, T., Fonagy, P., & Montague, P. R. (2008). The rupture and repair of cooperation in borderline personality disorder. *Science, 321*(5890), 806–810. https://doi.org/10.1126/science.1156902

Kobak, R. R., & Kerig, P. K. (2015). Introduction to the special issue: Attachment-based treatments for adolescents. *Attachment and Human Development, 17*(2), 111–118. https://doi.org/10.1080/14616734.2015.1006382

Krause, S., Pokorny, D., Schury, K., Doyen-Waldecker, C., Hulbert, A., Karabat-siakis, A., Kolassa, I., Gündel, G., Waller, C., & Buchheim, A. (2016). Effects of the adult attachment projective picture system on oxytocin and cortisol blood levels in mothers. *Frontiers in Human Neuroscience 10,* 627 [Online 8 December 2016, 2016. https://doi.org/10.3389/fnhum.2016.00627]

Lenhart, L., Gander, M., Steiger, R., Dabkowska-Mika, A., Mangesius, S., Haid-Stecher, N., Fuchs, M., Buchheim, A., Sevecke, K., & Gizewski, E. R. (2022). Attachment status is associated with grey matter recovery in adolescent anorexia nervosa: Findings from a longitudinal study *European Journal of Neuroscience.* [Epub ahead of print] https://doi.org/10.1111/ejn.15614.

Levy, K. N., Meehan, K. B., Kelly, K. M., Reynoso, J. S., Weber, M., Clarkin, J. F., & Kernberg, O. F. (2006). Change in attachment patterns and reflective function in a randomized control trial of transference-focused psychotherapy for borderline personality disorder. *Journal of Consulting and Clinical Psychology,* 74(6), 1027–1040. https://doi.org/10.1037/0022-006X.74.6.1027

Maxwell, H., Tasca, G. A., Grenon, R., Ritchie, K., Bissada, H., & Balfour, L. (2017). Change in attachment states of mind of women with binge-eating disorder. *Clinical Psychology and Psychotherapy,* 24(6), 1292–1303. https://doi.org/10.1002/cpp.2095

Slade, A. (2008). The implications of attachment theory and research for adult psychotherapy: Research and clinical perspectives. In J. Cassidy & P. R. Shaver (Eds.), *Handbook of attachment: Theory, research, and clinical applications* (2nd ed., pp. 762–782). Guilford Press.

Venta, A., Shmueli-Goetz, Y., & Sharp, C. (2014). Assessing attachment in adolescence: A psychometric study of the child attachment interview. *Psychological Assessment,* 26(1), 238–255. http://doi.org/10.1037/a0034712

Warmuth, K. A., & Cummings, E. M. (2015). Examining developmental fit of the adult attachment interview in adolescence. *Developmental Review, 36,* 200–218. https://doi.org/10.1016/j.dr.2015.04.002

Webster, L., & Joubert, D. (2011). Use of the adult attachment projective picture system in an assessment of an adolescent in foster care. *Journal of Personal Assessment,* 93(5), 417–426. https://doi.org/10.1080/00223891.2011.594127

Part 2

Incomplete pathological mourning

4 Attachment trauma and incomplete pathological mourning

Carol George

The dictionary defines trauma as a violently produced physical or psychological wound accompanied by shock (Webster's dictionary). In psychiatry, trauma is partly determined by the enduring emotional effects of shock and alarm, including chronic debilitating anxiety, fear, and anger. The attachment theory approach is narrower, beginning historically with Bowlby's discussion of loss (Bowlby, 1980; Main & Hesse, 1990; Main & Solomon, 1986). For over three decades, attachment trauma has been equated to loss and abuse, which researchers explored as the precursor for children's disorganized attachment and developmental and mental health risk, and brain functioning across the life span, as well as trauma later in life (Hughes et al., 2017; Marcusson-Clavertz et al., 2017; Schimmenti, 2022; Stovall-McClough & Dozier, 2016; Verhage et al., 2016). This chapter expands our view of attachment trauma and describes how to assess it using the Adult Attachment Projective Picture System (AAP).

Of particular interest to clinicians are individuals who show signs of trauma and have not experienced loss or abuse. Instead, they frequently describe non-catastrophic experiences, often called by clinicians little t trauma (e.g., divorce, emotional abuse, chronic parental misattunement). Little t trauma is legitimate trauma; from an attachment perspective, these experiences instinctively signal extreme danger. A study by Solomon and George (2011b) helps us think about the traumatic effects of these experiences on children's attachment. These researchers explored mothers' childhood backgrounds to determine why so many children with disorganized attachment in their study did not have mothers who reported loss or childhood maltreatment. Thinking about fear, they defined trauma as childhood life events that were "assaults to attachment," that is, frightening situations where children need protection. In addition to loss, these events included all forms of family violence, parental affect dysregulation (e.g., unpredictable uncontrollable negative affect), and substance abuse. Importantly, what predicted attachment disorganization was not the events themselves but the mothers' describing experiences of chronic parental "failed protection" or failed self-protection (i.e., the inability to take action to protect the self – see Chapter 1).

DOI: 10.4324/9781003215431-6

This failure creates a "toxic traumatic stress" reaction that undermines behavioral, representational, and neurophysiological regulation (Solomon & George, 2011a). Solomon and George (George & Solomon, 2011; Solomon & George, 2011b) emphasized that the mothers' experience in their study, and later representation, is characterized by dysregulating fear and feeling helpless and desperately alone. Consequently, failed protection by attachment figures, whether abusive or not, compromises psychological safety, self-integrity, and ultimately, survival. Children are left physically or psychologically abandoned in those frightening moments when they need protection the most. Indeed, the attachment figures themselves may be the children's source of fear (Main & Hesse, 1996). However, attachment trauma is not always that simple. Instead, trauma describes a broken attachment-caregiving relationship. Attachment and caregiving are neither working reciprocally nor are mutually informing. The parents themselves are profoundly helpless and behave in ways that threaten or leave their children vulnerable to threats by others or the environment. The origins of the parents' helplessness can be in their childhoods or the childrearing environments. A complete discussion of the etiology of failed protection and helplessness is beyond the scope of this chapter. Interested readers are referred to the work of George and Solomon (2008) describing parental caregiving.

Mourning attachment trauma

All attachment trauma, like loss, must be mourned. Past relationships must be revisited, at least at the representational level; painful affect must be integrated into current representations of self to achieve the emotional and relational resiliency and repair that completes the mourning process. When mourning is incomplete, the individuals consciously or unconsciously believe that trauma is still reversible (i.e. they can go back in time and undo the traumatic experience). Representational models of the self and the surrounding world remain unchanged. Bowlby (1980) explained that life is "planned on a false basis or else falls into unplanned disarray" (p. 138). Individuals remain in a "state of suspended growth in which [they are] held prisoner by the dilemma [they] cannot solve" (p. 139).

Bowlby (1980) described this psychological suspension as "pathological mourning." He used the term pathological because individuals who have not completed mourning exhibit seemingly never-ending signs of traumatic stress. Some avoid situations or memories reminiscent of the trauma at all costs to prevent triggering. Others describe invasions or becoming flooded by memories, affect, flashbacks, or distressing dreams. Individuals may become inexplicably angry or enraged, irritable, hypervigilant, and have trouble thinking clearly (which can mimic ADHD). They feel guilty (misattribution of self as the cause of trauma) and ashamed. Behavioral symptoms may include dissociation or self-destructive behavior (e.g., using drugs or alcohol in unhealthy ways). Pathological mourning also assaults relationships. Dysregulated affect and behavior can drive away even those in the closest relationships and compromise parenting a new generation of children. Pathological mourning compromises physical and mental health across the life span. Epigenetic researchers have shown how children inherit the biological and neurophysiological effects of their parents' attachment trauma (Krippner & Barrett, 2019).

Bowlby's (1980) description of the "healthy" (also termed "normal") course of mourning helps us understand pathological manifestations where individuals get stuck. The first phase of healthy mourning is numbness and shock, an adaptive stress response that allows individuals to orient toward events and prepare for action. After the shock wears off, individuals realize that the attachment figure is not accessible. The response to this knowledge activates the second phase of mourning. Similar to infants who are separated from their parents, the hallmark of this phase is yearning and searching for the "lost" attachment figure. In situations that do not involve death, searching for the attachment figure puts individuals in what seems to be an irresolvable situation. Physical availability does not ensure psychological accessibility, basic care, or parental sensitivity. Every search risks a devastating reminder of attachment figure abdication. Under these conditions, a reunion is impossible. The result is plunging into the third phase of mourning, described by Bowlby as a state of "disorganization and despair." This phase is also characterized by intense anger. Again, like separated infants, individuals are also angry that their search was unsuccessful. They may also be angry at themselves (reproach, shame) as the result of attributions that they did not do anything or enough to prevent the loss (survivor's guilt). They typically reject others who they view as failing to help them complete their search. Individuals may also be angry at the lost attachment figure for abandoning them. "Completion" of the mourning process requires a cognitive-emotional reorganization of individuals' representations of the attachment figure and the self. They must be able to "see" and "name" traumatic events; most importantly, they must recognize what it means when parents failed to protect them and that their parents' failure was not their fault. In sum, completing the mourning process restructures the representation of the self. The end goal is to recognize a changed self living in changed circumstances and revise their attachment model to be a coherent reflection of the present in light of the past. Only then can individuals redefine their life goals. There is a fine line between the healthy and pathological course of mourning, and completion depends partly on defensive processes. Mourning is not completed when defenses are rigid and restrict or take over mental functioning.

There is no specified time frame to complete mourning for loss. There are cultural practices that can help individuals stay on course (e.g., placement of the headstone one year following a loss; Bowlby, 1980; Parkes, 2006). Many people do not begin grieving even severe trauma after several years have passed. Pathological mourning is indicated when individuals show no signs of improving. Some individuals remain confused about the source of their maladies or distress, complaints, or behavior that others may deem irrational. Others show deteriorating mental or physical health.

Bowlby (1980) described three variations of pathological mourning. One is the prolonged absence of grieving or Failed Mourning, which extends prolonged shock and numbing. Grieving never begins. Realizing that they cannot reverse the trauma is too painful and terrifying to dwell on. Deactivating defenses (see Chapter 1) shift the Failed Mourner's attention and behavior away from or attempt to neutralize painful reminders of the trauma. The trauma may be "so ill-defined and remote from consciousness that much therapeutic work [is needed] to make it manifest" (Bowlby, 1980, p. 141). Individuals engage in what they consider an everyday life and take pride in carrying on as if nothing had happened. They are involved, efficient, and appear to the external world to be coping well. This presentation can take the form of *compulsive self-reliance*. Self-sufficient, individuals do not reach out to or seek comfort from others. They are proud of their independence and self-control, despise sentimentality, and view crying as a sign of weakness (Bowlby, 1980, p. 153). These responses are all emotion regulation strategies to lock away anger, pain, and sorrow.

Some Failed Mourners become *compulsive caregivers* who seek out others to care for. Their caregiving behavior, however, lacks empathy and interpersonal attunement. Instead, compulsive caregiving is a self-care strategy driven by their unconscious hope that caring for others will bring them comfort. And for a while, caring for others may succeed in bringing them comfort, but this comfort evaporates as negative affect leaks in. Understandably, compulsive caregiving is often directed to others who have experienced trauma. Caregiving is centered on their own needs and can become an obsession. Relationships are at risk of becoming complicated by possessiveness and jealousy, believing that the cared-for is having such an easy time (Lehmann, personal communication, April 6, 2021). Resentment also builds up because their longing to be taken care of is cut off and buried deep inside. So not only are Failed Mourners jealous, but they can also start to resent the fact that they are not getting the same care in return.

Individuals naturally yearn and search for missing attachment figures when the numbness wears off. When this happens, individuals move into variations of incomplete mourning that Bowlby (1980) termed *chronic mourning*. Hence, some individuals begin the mourning process and get stuck in a chronic mourning state that centers around an impossible search to reunite with the attachment figure. Reunion with attachment figures who are dead or abdicate caregiving is doomed for failure. This failure is devastating; chronic mourning is unusually intense and prolonged. Individuals cannot replan their lives and cannot find comfort in others. Anger, self-blame, guilt, shame, and feelings of worthlessness dominate and persist, but without evidence of sorrow and sadness. Individuals show varying degrees of depression and anxiety. There is still a glimmer of hope that trauma is reversible; realizing this is impossible creates stress, frustration, and pain.

There can be different paths to chronic mourning. Some individuals move through the grieving process and end up "stuck" in chronic mourning. Bowlby (1980) also described how individuals in Failed Mourning are at risk of plunging into a chronic mourning state when their deactivating defenses break down or they experience another trauma.

Chronic mourning takes two forms. One is Preoccupied with Personal Suffering, which Bowlby (1980) viewed as a defensive distortion of yearning and searching; the defense involved is cognitive disconnection (see Chapter 1). Individuals become overwhelmed, frightened, hypervigilant, and mentally preoccupied with trauma. Disconnecting defenses create an illusion of survival by diffusing the details of traumatic events and making a conscious fog. It is as if preoccupied sufferers survive trauma by not "knowing" what happened to them. What they do know, however, is that they are terrified and in pain. Preoccupied sufferers report high levels of distress and are depressed and anxious. They are unable to articulate the painful historical details of their traumatic experiences or explain why they feel unprotected and afraid. For some, these feelings often give way to sadness, longing for attachment figures, and sentimental sorrow. Endlessly yearning and searching, like the ambivalent-resistant infant, they can become angry or enraged. In sum, disconnection may prevent them from feeling helpless and slipping into disorganization but robs them of the agency needed to grieve and complete mourning. George and West (2012) described this affective state as "living in the war zone."

The other form is Unresolved mourning, which is an extension of the disorganization and despair phase of healthy mourning.[1] Main and her colleagues (Hesse, 2016; Main & Goldwyn, 1985–2003) described Unresolved mourning for loss as the underlying disbelief that the person is dead. Unresolved mourning creates doubt that events occurred or were even traumatic. This mental state is often accompanied by feeling responsible for the trauma and an inability to consider other causes. Individuals become disoriented in space and time, psychologically confused, or try to undo or erase the experiences. Some unresolved mourners go into "gory" detail or become eulogistic. Defenses are broken (George & West, 2012). Neither defensive deactivation nor disconnection can prevent individuals from becoming flooded or overwhelmed. Instead, the trauma remains fresh and uncontained.

Assessing pathological mourning and trauma risk using the AAP

Bowlby's (1980) tripartite model of mourning unifies our conceptualization of the process of grieving attachment trauma, and the AAP coding system identifies the current risk for pathological mourning. The AAP is the only attachment assessment that provides clinicians with a means to assess this tripartite model of attachment trauma and trace changes in the grieving process when used in long-term psychotherapy.

The AAP trauma coding system originated during the author's collaboration with Dr. Anna Buchheim on a study of psychiatric patients at high risk for relationship-based trauma (e.g., Borderline Personality Disorder, anxiety disorder, Post-Traumatic Stress Disorder; Buchheim & George, 2011). We noticed variations in the intensity of the segregated systems described in patients' stories (see Chapter 1). We also noticed stories that included unusual, surreal, or disturbing material differing from response material defined as segregated systems. Indeed, the history of attachment assessment has benefited from paying attention to what "does not fit." For example, attending to perplexing infant behavior in the Strange Situation, such as freezing or hiding during the reunion with the parent, led to the disorganized child attachment classification (George & Main, 1979; Main & Solomon, 1986).

Concerning segregated systems, some AAP story themes seemed "normative" (pulled for by the picture) and benign. For example, the Cemetery scene pulls for *speaking to the deceased*. Another example is feeling *frightened* by a nightmare in response to Bed. By comparison, other stories, such as this Corner story, were terrifying.[2]

> It's a little kid... in the corner... begging somebody to stop... possibly *hitting* him. And he looks *scared*. The kid did nothing; this is all on the grownup trying to *hit* this kid. Maybe they were angry, maybe they *drank*, maybe due to *substance, abuse,* or other... you know, other personal issues. But this kid is definitely *afraid* and hoping that it would stop. The kid is *afraid* and upset, and *betrayed*. It's too much, and the grownup is for some reason, angry. And *taking it out on this little kid*. Maybe blaming the little kid for something that the kid couldn't have possibly been blamed for. It's a horrible picture.

In addition to attachment trauma, we evaluated narratives for odd or unusual story material that provided evidence of an individual's risk for derealization. Derealization describes the characters or surroundings as somehow unreal, sometimes created by descriptions of "out-of-the-world" experiences or images associated with the threat of self-fragmentation in the absence of protection from trauma (Cook et al., 2017; Lerner, 1998). These stories had elements that reminded us of the lapses of reality described by severely abused individuals who cope by "leaving the self." We were not surprised to discover in retrospect that these individuals had indeed experienced extreme attachment trauma, such as chronic sexual abuse or life threats. The coding system specified five derealization dimensions. The first, surreal, is most common. This material describes the character as not grounded in the real world, such as wanting to be in outer space, floating above the bench, having a seizure, or the undead rising from the grave. The other dimensions include absorbed withdrawal, such as wanting to be invisible; evil-sinister, such as a caregiver who cannot wait to do "evil" things to a child; disgust-contempt, such as severe shaming by telling the child that he is disgusting or dumb and worthless; and sexual, such as pornography or oblique descriptions suggesting sexual violation (e.g., the girl is naked from the waist down; the boy does not want to see those nasty pictures).

The next step after developing the trauma coding system was to validate it. The validation process used the Adult Attachment Interview (AAI, George et al., 1984; Main & Goldwyn, 1985–2003), the same interviews used in the original AAP validation study (George & West, 2012). The AAI only asks about individuals' experiences with loss and abuse, so empirical validation addressed the question of whether the AAP could identify pathological mourning for those experiences. The AAIs that included loss or abuse experiences were classified into three pathological mourning groups.[3] Failed Mourning is not an established AAI classification group. It was identified using the Hamilton-Oravetz and George rating scale for Failed Mourning (Hamilton-Oravetz, 1993) and appears as a mentally "armored" subgroup of Dismissing attachment. Preoccupation with personal suffering is a traumatized disconnected subgroup and identified using Main's criteria for the trauma subgroup of the Preoccupied classification (Hesse, 2016; Main & Goldwyn, 1985–2003). Unresolved attachment is an established AAI classification. Discriminant analyses demonstrated a significant correspondence between the AAP and AAI for pathological mourning groups for loss and abuse.[4] Misses may have been partly because the AAI does not pursue other forms of trauma. In addition, the AAP may be more trauma sensitive than the AAI because the AAP never asks individuals to tell their personal stories (Jones-Mason, personal communication, August 10, 2010).

Clinicians increasingly attest to the central role of identifying pathological mourning in their assessment reports and psychotherapy. Clinicians and researchers alike report that individuals who experienced loss or abuse are also likely to describe other forms of trauma (e.g., Murphy et al., 2014). As noted, the AAP is not a biographical interview; it reveals the hypothetical stories of clients' lives. Clinicians often learn of clients' real traumas through psychotherapy or other assessments. It is recommended that researchers use a trauma interview with the AAP to uncover unnamed loss or abuse or other forms of traumatic failed protection. Without a trauma interview, therapists who are not working long term with clients will miss out on uncovering essential experiences. Some therapists prefer getting access to memories using the Early Memories Procedure (EMP, Bruhn, 1992) that do not put clients on the spot to describe trauma. Many clients do not want to identify as "traumatized." The EMP is an excellent way to access memories of failed protection.

Conclusion

Theory building and the clinical application of attachment trauma are limited by a long-standing tradition in attachment theory that confines trauma as experiences of loss or abuse. Yet we know the role that other traumatic life events and failed protection play in our clients' lives and how these experiences are sources of debilitating shock, distress, and fear. This chapter demonstrated reconceptualizing attachment trauma in terms of parental abdication and failed protection and aligns clinicians with implementing the full spectrum of Bowlby's thinking about grief and mourning. The AAP provides the field for the first time in the history of attachment with a developmental assessment of attachment trauma risk that circumvents the pitfalls of self-report measures. Many of the cases in this book involve clients with pathological mourning and discussions of assessment outcomes and treatment recommendations.

Notes

1 Bowlby never used the term Unresolved to describe this form of mourning. The term was applied to incomplete mourning of loss by Main and colleagues (1985).
2 Bold = trauma.
3 The designation of the AAP pathological groups requires training and is beyond the scope of this chapter. Classifications have demonstrated inter-judge reliability with significant agreement Kappa's, $p < 0.001$.
4 The correct classification rate was 68% for the AAI-Ds group differentiations; 13/15 dismissing cases and 10/18 Failed Mourning were correctly classified ($X^2 = 11.90$, $p < 0.001$). The correct classification rate was 83% for the AAI-E group differentiations; 17/19 Preoccupied and 7/10 Preoccupied with Personal Suffering cases were correctly classified ($X^2 = 18.37$, $p < 0.001$). The correct classification rate was 92% for AAI-Unresolved group differentiations; 23/24 Resolved and 22/25 complicated grief cases were correctly classified ($X^2 = 37.97$, $p < 0.001$).

References

Bowlby, J. (1973). *Attachment and loss: Vol. 2. Separation: Anxiety and anger.* Basic Books.

Bowlby, J. (1980). *Attachment and loss: Vol. 3. Loss: Sadness and depression.* Basic Books.

Bruhn, A. R. (1992). The early memories procedure: A projective test of autobiographical memory: I. *Journal of Personality Assessment, 58*(1), 1–15 https://doi.org/10.1207/s15327752jpa5801_1

Buchheim, A., & George, C. (2011). The representational, neurobiological, and emotional foundation of attachment disorganization in borderline personality disorder and anxiety disorder. In J. Solomon & C. George (Eds.), *Disorganization of attachment and caregiving* (pp. 343–382). Guilford Press.

Cook, A., Spinazzola, J., Ford, J. Lanktree, C., Blaustein, M., Cloitre, M., & van der Kolk, B. (2017). Complex trauma in children and adolescents. *Psychiatric Annals, 35*(5), 390–398. https://doi.org/10.3928.00485713-20050501-05

George, C., Kaplan, N., & Main, M. (1984). *The Adult Attachment Interview* [In Unpublished Doctoral Dissertation, University of California], Berkeley, CA.

George, C., & Main, M. (1979). Social interactions of young abused children: Approach, avoidance, and aggression. *Child Development, 50*(2), 306–318. https://doi.org/10.2307/1129405

George, C., & Solomon, J. (2011). Caregiving helplessness: The development of a screening measure for disorganized maternal caregiving. In J. Solomon & C. George (Eds.), *Disorganized attachment and caregiving* (pp. 133–163). Guilford Press.

George, C., & West, M. (2012). *The adult attachment projective picture system: Attachment theory and assessment in adults.* Guilford Press.

Hamilton-Oravetz, S. (1993). *Patterns of attachment and grief in primary care medicine patients* [Unpublished doctoral dissertation]. California School for Professional Psychology, Berkeley, CA

Hesse, E. (2016). The Adult Attachment Interview: Protocol, method of analysis, and selected empirical studies: 1985–2015. In J. Cassidy & P. Shaver (Eds.), *Handbook of attachment: Theory, research, and clinical applications* (pp. 553–597). Guilford Press.

Hughes, K., Bellis, M. A., Hardcastle, K. A., Sethi, D., Butchart, A. Mikton, C., & Dunne, M. P. (2017). The effect of multiple adverse childhood experiences on health: A systematic review and meta-analysis. *The Lancet. Public Health,* e356–e366. https://doi.org/10.1016/S2468-2667(17)30118-4

Krippner, S., & Barrett, D. (2019). Transgenerational trauma: The role of epigenetics. *Journal of Mind and Behavior, 40*(1), 53–62.

Lerner, P. (1998). *Psychoanalytic perspectives on the Rorschach.* Analytic Press.

Main, M., & Goldwyn, R. (1985–2003). *Adult attachment scoring and classification system* [Unpublished rating and classification manual]. University of California, Berkeley, CA

Main, M., & Hesse, E. (1990). Parents' unresolved traumatic experiences are related to infant disorganized attachment status: Is frightened and/or frightening parental behavior the linking mechanism? In M. T. Greenberg, D. Cicchetti, & E. M. Cummings (Eds.), *Attachment in the preschool years* (pp. 161–182). University of Chicago Press.

Main, M., & Solomon, J. (1986). Discovery of a new, insecure disorganized/disoriented attachment pattern. In T. B. Brazelton & M. Yogman (Eds.), *Affective development in infancy* (pp. 95–124). Ablex.

Marcusson-Clavertz, D., Gušić, S., Bengtsson, H., Jacobsen, H., & Cardeña, E. (2017). The relation of dissociation and mind wandering to unresolved/disorganized attachment: an experience sampling study. *Attachment and Human Development, 19*(2), 170–190. https://doi.org/10.1080/14616734.2016.1261914

Murphy, A., Steele, M., Dube, S. R., Bate, J., Bonuck, K., Meissner, P., Goldman, H., & Steele, H. (2014). Adverse childhood experiences (ACEs) questionnaire and adult attachment interview (AAI): Implications for parent-child relationships. *Child Abuse and Neglect, 38*(2), 224–233. https://doi.org/10.1016/j.chiabu.2013.09.004

Parkes, C. M. (2006). *Love and loss: The roots of grief and its complications.* Routledge.

Schimmenti, A. (2022). The aggressor within: Attachment trauma, segregated systems, and the double face of shame. In O. B. Epstien (Ed.) *Shame matters: Attachment and relational perspectives for psychotherapists.* Routledge.

Solomon, J., & George, C. (2011a). The disorganized attachment-caregiving system: Dysregulation of adaptive processes at multiple levels. In J. Solomon & C. George (Eds.), *Disorganized attachment and caregiving* (pp. 3–24). Guilford Press.

Solomon, J., & George, C. (2011b). Dysregulation of maternal caregiving across two generations. In J. Solomon & C. George (Eds.), *Disorganization of attachment and caregiving* (pp. 25–51). Guilford Press.

Stovall-McClough, K. C., & Dozier, M. (2016). Attachment states of mind and psychopathology in adulthood. In J. Cassidy & P. R. Shaver (Eds.), *Handbook of attachment: Theory, research, and clinical implications* (3rd ed., pp. 715–738). Guilford Press.

Verhage, M. L., Schuengel, C., Madigan, S., Fearon, R. M. P., Oosterman, M., Cassibba, R., Bakermans-Kranenburg, M. J., & van IJzendoorn, M. H. (2016). Narrowing the transmission gap: A synthesis of three decades of research on intergenerational transmission of attachment. *Psychological Bulletin, 142*(4), 337–366. https://doi.org/10.1037/bul0000038

5 Failed Mourning

The sounds of silence

Melissa Lehmann

Attachment, trauma, grief, and mourning are central to human biology. Bowlby (1982) defined attachment as a biologically based behavioral system that drives us instinctively to stay close to our attachment figures for protection and survival. Our biology defines what is traumatic (e.g., Perry et al., 1995; Van Der Kolk, 2006). The primitive parts of our brain "know" and remember what is dangerous, frightening, and threatening well before we have the words to describe our feelings (Perry et al., 1995). We fight, flee, or freeze before we consciously register what is happening (Perry et al., 1995). Grieving the loss or absence of someone we love is also an innate characteristic of humans and primates alike. When attachment figures die or attachment relationships are broken, we are biologically driven to grieve the emotional disturbance that follows in order to re-establish physiological and emotional equilibrium. If we are prevented from doing this, then cognitive, physical, and emotional problems ensue. The failure to grieve then is a loss of self (Bowlby, 1980; Parkes, 2006).

Bowlby (1980) described the evolutionary function of mourning the death of an attachment figure and what happens when the grief process is interrupted (see Chapter 4). Following this line of thinking, contemporary attachment theorists extended Bowlby's ideas regarding loss through death to include all forms of attachment trauma where attachment figures abdicated their protective role leaving children frightened, helpless, and having to fend for themselves (George & Solomon, 2008; George & West, 2012; Solomon & George, 1996). This view emphasizes that our instinctual need to grieve is not limited to death and extends to experiences of caregiver emotional unavailability and failure to respond in those critical moments when children are the most distressed. George and West (2012) emphasized that early experiences of caregiver failure to assuage attachment distress and help children regulate mind, body, and emotions lie at the heart of attachment trauma. These failures, regardless of the reason, interfere with the ability to understand painful experience, feel and express frightening emotion, and interrupt the grief process that is necessary for emotional balance and well-being. The inability to mourn such attachment failures prevents us from being able

DOI: 10.4324/9781003215431-7

to integrate these experiences into our lives and leaves us haunted by feelings of confusion, fear, rage, shame, and emptiness (Bowlby, 1980; Frumkin et al., 2021).

This chapter highlights how the Adult Attachment Projective Picture System (AAP) was the tool that allowed the author to identify the client's attachment trauma and the defensive processes he used to protect himself against it. The case example presents the journey of a 47-year-old Failed Mourner during a Therapeutic Assessment (Finn, 2007) and illuminates how the AAP helped this client for the first time be able to see and acknowledge his early attachment experiences with his attachment figures as traumatic. The AAP shows the ways in which this Failed Mourner learned to guard against his feelings of pain and the costs of being blocked from mourning his caregivers' ongoing failed protection and emotional unavailability. The chapter ends with a discussion of how one might talk to their clients about attachment, the AAP results, and the concept of Failed Mourning.

Failed Mourning: The sounds of silence

Failed Mourning, or as Bowlby (1980) termed it the *prolonged absence of grieving*, speaks for itself. The grief process has been blocked; mourning fails because it never begins. For Failed Mourners, life continues as if nothing happened. Defensive deactivation constitutes the core of Failed Mourning, it creates an illusion of safety and security because it armors individuals against dysregulating affect by shutting out the details and perceptions of traumatic experiences and their associated fear, anger, shame, and sadness. Trauma is silenced. There is nothing to grieve. Like Paul Simon's song *The Sound of Silence* (Simon et al., 2001), Failed Mourners walk in the echoes of the sounds of their silenced childhoods.

Failed Mourning is a form of incomplete pathological mourning that manifests as Dismissing attachment (see Chapter 4). Its origins lie in Avoidant childhood attachment. George and Solomon (2008) observed that Avoidant attachment is built on relational distance, functional care (taking care of the problem without addressing emotional distress), and an emphasis on independence and intellectual achievement at the expense of caregiving sensitivity, intimacy, and mutual enjoyment. Negative affect is downplayed or rejected, for example, in parental reproaches such as "don't cry" and "there is nothing to fear." Anger is uncomfortable and risks punishment and labeling children as misbehaving, manipulative, or uncooperative. The Avoidant child camouflages their negative affect as well as their caregiver's negative affect and rejection of their attachment needs by creating an ideal representation of attachment figures as caring, supportive, involved, and loving (Solomon et al., 1995). The Avoidant child appears outwardly strong, independent, and calm (Solomon et al., 1995). Emotional care is not on their radar, and avoidance guards against painful emotions, rejection, and vulnerability (Hesse, 2016).

What happens when these children experience trauma? Deactivating defenses that maintain emotional and relational distance work on overdrive (George & West, 2012). Their avoidant shell becomes fortified and controlling their internal and external worlds becomes the major life task. This process becomes the foundation upon which the Failed Mourner stands. There is no one to turn to except the self. They cannot speak of what their parents will not speak. If spoken, no one listens, no one hears. They cannot acknowledge what their parents will not acknowledge. They cannot feel or express their sadness, anger, or pain because their parents do not tolerate these emotions. *They silence their grief because they are silenced.*

The Failed Mourner is left alone with no one to help them remember, share their feelings, or "hold" them while they grieve. They must block all conscious remembrance of their attachment figure's failed protection and continue on in life. The dilemma, however, is that the trauma, anguish, and pain still remain. They do not vanish into the darkness of the mind but instead become the seeds upon which the self is organized. As time passes, the inevitable leakage of these past experiences comes to take hold in a way that greatly impacts the Failed Mourner's emotional state and relational world. Representations of normal caregiving relationships and an ideal childhood backfire (Bowlby, 1980), confusion sets in, and the Failed Mourner is left asking "*WHY* do I feel this way when I have no reason to feel this way?"

Our clients often enter our rooms asking why. They are desperate for some kind of rational explanation for why they feel the way they feel, besides just feeling that something is fundamentally wrong with them. This is where the AAP becomes an irreplaceable tool. Its unique ability to assess attachment trauma and the defenses used to protect against it provides us with a way to help our clients see and understand why they feel and act the way they do, and where their struggles with intimacy and human connection began. The AAP stories give words to what has been unspoken. It validates our clients' experiences by naming them and helps reduce the shame they have carried with them for so long. The AAP counters their self-evaluations of being bad, wrong, or damaged beyond repair, for there is a reason they feel the way they do. In short, the AAP validates our clients' attachment trauma.

This is exactly where I met Ethan when he walked into my room a few years ago – looking for answers, searching for understanding and validation. He hoped that a Therapeutic Assessment would explain his history of depression and anxiety, distraction and inattention, and feelings of blankness and detachment from the world around him.

Ethan: The journey of a Failed Mourner

At the time of the assessment, Ethan was 46 years old and had been married for 15 years. He was and is a highly successful graphic designer with a long list of accomplishments. He had been in and out of therapy since the age of 20 and on medication for depression and anxiety for over 18 years. He described periods in his life where he felt okay and then times when he said he would crash or collapse. He said he felt stuck and did not know what to do to feel better. He said he wanted to be happy. When I inquired about the last time he felt happy, he replied after a long silence, "it has been a long time."

Ethan pinpointed his crashes as occurring after break-ups and more recently when he was overwhelmed by the thought of his marriage ending. The threat to his marriage meant being alone – being isolated, which Bowlby (1982) explained as the most excruciating of primate experiences, even worse than death. He was terrified and willing to go to great lengths to avoid this from happening. During times of separation from his wife, he would immerse himself in his work to avoid feeling anxious and depressed. This deactivating strategy worked for him for a while, but over time, feelings of emptiness and despair would take hold, leaving him feeling like "a blank person."

Looking back to Ethan's childhood, his school experience was agonizing. It was marred by hostility (bullying and ridicule), isolation (always feeling alone), and shame (feeling stupid for not doing well in school, his mom yelling and calling him spacey when he would forget to do something). He described how he still struggles with distraction and how this has been an ongoing area of contention between him and his wife. Ethan reported that he was unable to focus or concentrate when he and his wife argued and that afterward he had difficulty remembering what occurred. He was able to identify his anxiety at these times, as well as his discomfort with his wife's anger. Anger left him feeling as if he had done something wrong, which led to him having to defend himself or withdrawing and crumbling into a place of shame and self-criticism.

Ethan's description of his childhood was filled with murky and conflicting evaluations of his upbringing, which is not uncommon for many clients when they first enter our rooms. He described his childhood as "relatively normal," but he also felt his parents never understood him. He described his mom as "sweet" but full of contradictions. When asked to elaborate, he said that she often presented herself as "laid back" but was in fact highly anxious. The image of his father was also confusing. Ethan described him as "sweet but unemotional," except when it came to his temper. Throughout his life, Ethan had witnessed his father "erupt." Although his father was never physically abusive, his rages were unpredictable, and Ethan said he was frightened and confused because there was no apparent reason for him to be so angry. End all be all, Ethan summed up the description of his parents as supportive just "not really emotional people."

These descriptions demonstrate how hard Ethan was trying to make sense of his early experiences. His semantic description of an ideal normal childhood contradicted the murky images and depictions of his parents that were not so "sweet." As he tried to hold on to an "ideal" representation of his childhood, he was plagued with confusion and uncertainty regarding his emotional state, his relationships and the "gaping hole" he felt inside. Ethan's questions for the assessment exemplify the place he was in when he first came to see me, as well as his knowing that something else was there. Something that he had been unable to see because he had not been allowed to see it. His question, *Do I have a wall? And if so, what is it guarding?* speaks directly to this awareness.

Ethan's testing: What do we see?

We did four tests together: MMPI-2, Rorschach, the AAP, and Early Memories Procedure (EMP). This chapter focuses on the intersection of the AAP with the MMPI-2 and Rorschach.

MMPI-2

The MMPI-2 is a self-report measure that depicts how a client sees himself and his self-awareness. Ethan's MMPI-2 results were fraught with pain and anguish. Many of the clinical scales were elevated above the clinical cutoff. His self-report told me directly how awful he felt and that he did not know why or what to do about it. The results (code-type 2–7–8) spoke to his relentless depression and self-hatred, as well as the unbearable tension he had been living with for so many years (Caldwell, 2008). The results also told me that he felt stuck and hopeless, that he lacked confidence in interpersonal relationships, and that he did not have adequate resources to cope with the intensity of his emotional distress. In other words, "life is awful, and I can't do anything about it." His MMPI-2 suggested that he had no access to anger or the ability to assert or protect himself. His cutoff anger seemed to manifest as depression and self-criticism. The results also showed initial signs of trauma and his dismissal of attachment issues. His PK scale, a scale developed to identify veterans with PTSD that signifies extreme emotional distress, was elevated. On the other hand, his Family Problems Content scale was not elevated, which spoke to the idealized normal childhood image he was holding onto in his conscious mind. Although neither of these findings are evidential on their own, they help set the stage for interpreting the AAP.

Rorschach: What lies below

Ethan's Rorschach gives us a more nuanced look at the MMPI-2 findings, adding a level of complexity and depth to what he was able to say directly about himself. One nuance that emerged from the Rorschach was the variability in Ethan's ability to cope and manage life. Ethan had said that he could cope at times, and this is exactly what his Rorschach showed. When his life is running smoothy, and he can focus, has structure, and is free of emotional duress, Ethan seems to do quite well. His abundance of navigational resources – intelligence, creativity, reasoning, and a logical mind help create a sense of feeling fine when there are no bumps in his life. But this is not the entire story. The Rorschach also told a story of the other times, the times Ethan had alluded to as his crashes, the times he was so aptly able to describe in his self-report measure.

The Rorschach provided a window to see that these collapses tended to occur within the context of stressful relationships and when he was emotionally aroused. These events seemed to undermine his ability to cope and manage life on his own, which led to him collapsing in pain and despair. The Rorschach validated what he told me about break-ups and threats to his marriage being the precipitants of his crashes and showed a similar picture as to what he described on his MMPI-2. The results from the Rorschach also indicated that when Ethan collapses his view of self and world become distorted, he cannot trust what he perceives is happening around him. His ability to engage in self-reflection and his reliance upon his good thinking abilities become problematic at these times, for all he can see is someone who is damaged and broken. His emotional landscape becomes filled with shame, lack of self-worth, and a substantial amount of anger hidden from the outside world and turned in on himself.

Ethan's responses to the Rorschach also encompassed a host of traumatic material, fortifying the initial indications of trauma and extreme emotional distress shown on his MMPI-2. His Critical Content index was in the 99th percentile and his Trauma Content Index (TCI) was significantly elevated. His TCI was actually higher than the mean TCI of individuals who reported sexual abuse (Kamphuis et al., 2000), thus suggesting that he was in the same amount of emotional distress as someone who had been sexually abused. Although Ethan had no history of sexual or physical abuse, no neglect, and no other kind of Big T trauma, it was clear from his testing that he had in fact experienced significant trauma.

The MMPI-2 and Rorschach revealed the depth of Ethan's pain and emotional turmoil, what his crashes entail, and when they are most likely to occur; however, these assessments did not address the question of why these experiences were occurring. The puzzle around Ethan's emotional state, crashes, and significant signs of trauma still remained. The AAP had the answers to these questions and became the backbone for my understanding of Ethan and the work we would do together.

Ethan's AAP: Here within lies the WHY

Ethan's AAP showed the silence and darkness of his internal world. It gave words to that which had not been spoken, to the experiences and feelings he knew were there but was unable to acknowledge. His stories brought meaning and understanding to the results of the other two assessments. His Failed Mourning AAP classification became the cornerstone upon which we began to shift the perspective from "something is wrong with me" to "I experienced trauma and had to *learn* to survive."

Ethan's AAP is a tale of two worlds. One is buried deep inside; it is a world of isolation, fear, helplessness, shame, and the failed protection of his childhood. This is the world of attachment trauma. The other is his protective deactivation structure, the defensive shell he built to block conscious awareness of traumatic attachment affect. The function of this shell is to guard against the leakage of Ethan's unbearable feelings and fear that has been segregated and dismissed in order for him to survive and function in the world. The problem with this duality is attachment stress threatens the defensive shell and Failed Mourners risk facing an overwhelming landslide of painful emotion and traumatic experiences (Bowlby, 1980). The buried self breaks through and the individual faces devastation, confusion, and frightening isolation. Ethan's representational duality was most vividly evident in his AAP stories.

Alone stories

Ethan's alone stories tell the following narrative: "I am isolated, afraid, and helpless. I deactivate to create a shell that protects me *enough* to regulate on my own." It is striking that his alone stories are void of attachment figures or other people who could provide emotional support, care, or protection. The projected self faces shame, fear, confusion, and distress alone. His logical mind and achievement-oriented drive create the protective defensive shell. These deactivating processes help him manage his emotions and stop the leakage of his traumatic past.

His Bench story is a perfect example of this representational duality of his emotional worlds. The images in Bench denote his two worlds – the one that has been segregated and the one that protects him.

Here's a someone. She's upset and crying. My first instinct is to put her in a school setting. She's feeling incredibly sad, I think being *rejected*. That's feeling into a sense of being	Deactivate
isolated or **ostracized** from her peers. It's a *school setting.*	Trauma
She's getting *bullied by a peer in front of people in the*	Deactivate
lunchroom and she's gone outside to get away from everyone	Disconnect
and cry in private. She's sad, **ostracized, ashamed** that it	Traumatic
happened in front of other people. She's *thinking of options*	shame
if there's a way to not be in the situation. Maybe change	Deactivate
schools or think of other ways to fix the situation or thinking	Deactivate
she could have said in retrospect to combat a bully. She has	
to get herself out of there, collected, and go back to *class* and	Deactivate
hope that **no one notices she's been crying.**	Traumatic
	shame

This story shows how deactivation builds a shell around traumatizing feelings of isolation and shame. It protects Ethan enough so that he can start to use his logical mind to problem-solve his way out of this painful situation (thinking about options). Notice the absence of protective people. He is bullied, alone, ostracized, and ashamed. This is the essence of attachment trauma – failed protection on the part of his caregivers to provide safety and help him regulate (George & Solomon, 2008). He must protect himself, which means block his trauma out of his mind so he can go forward. At the end of the story narrative, he added, "I just got really sleepy which is a, sometimes a defense mechanism like if I want to avoid things I get really tired." Ethan's story and his self-reflection converge; both describe how he deactivates to manage and avoid thinking about his traumatic past and the overwhelming feelings in order to survive.

Ethan's response to the Corner picture, the most activating and stressful picture in the AAP sequence, provides an even clearer picture of this representational duality. His commentary while he narrates the story shows his conscious struggle to make sense of his trauma. The commentary is shown in the story in bold font.[1]

So it looks like he's trying not to be *hit* in a very weird	Trauma
corner. He's trying to keep from being *slapped*, he's	Trauma
trying to avoid physical harm, trying to avoid being hit.	
It seems like whatever **punishment it is unnecessary.**	Deactivate
Maybe the **parents have been drinking.** I mean it's	Trauma
hard for me to not as I'm saying these things reflect on	
what this is saying about myself and why I go to certain	
assumptions, wondering do I need to clarify in myself	
as to if the parents seem abusive from drinking. It's	
like, I've never, you know, my parents have never had	
drinking issues. So that's what led up to the parent being	
irrational. He seems *resigned to the situation, they're*	Trauma,
helpless to stop it. At this point they are just trying to	Disconnect
<u>protect</u> themselves the best they can and *biding their*	Agency: action
time until they can get out of the situation. You would	Disconnect
hope that the parent has some reflection on what they're	Disconnect
doing is *irrational* and they would come to their senses.	Trauma
It's more of a parent makes an empty *threat* and they're	Trauma,
biding their time until the parent calms down and *drinks*	Disconnect
themselves unconscious, but they get in the corner and	Trauma
<u>protect</u> themselves and eventually it's going to, they'll	Agency: action
wear themselves out or the threat will dissipate.	Disconnect

The narrative shows how he struggles to find a way to neutralize (i.e., deactivate) his fear and helplessness and his portrayal of a threatening out of control parent. He interrupts the narrative seeking a rational explanation for what appears to him to be irrational. This portrayal must mean there is something wrong with him. Unable to integrate his recalled normal childhood with the horror story he created exacerbates his shame.

We often write what we call an "attachment plot" that transforms the AAP story about hypothetical characters into the language of attachment theory. Ethan's attachment plot is, "My attachment figure is dangerously out of control. I am threatened, frightened, and helpless. No one protects me, so I must deactivate and protect myself." BUT underneath his deactivated shell, Ethan shows how frightened, alone, helpless, and ashamed he feels. Rather than accept the threat he describes, Ethan dismisses it as irrational and tells us that he believes "something must be wrong with me for feeling this way." This is the story of Failed Mourning. It shows Ethan's representational duality. The rational and irrational collide when the duality hits conscious processing, and he hears what he is saying about the parents in his story. His deactivated rational self (what he has learned and been told) successfully squelches his traumatic past, at least for the time being.

Dyadic stories

Ethan's dyadic stories connote an overriding sense of aloneness. His representation of *self* in such relationships is embedded in disconnected defenses. He becomes confused about his relationships particularly as he narrates how the attachment figure in his stories does not respond to his cues. He portrays attachment figures as insensitive, deactivated, and devastated to the extent that they fail to provide him with the comfort he needs even when he directly asks for it. All three dyadic stories show once again how he must rely on his own resources to regulate attachment distress. As when he is alone, he deactivates.

Ethan's Bed story illustrates the dyadic interaction that leads to the creation of the deactivating shell in response to caregiver insensitivity.[2]

A child seeks attention * from a parent at bedtime or the middle of the night. It looks like she's not as receptive to the request for attention from the child.	* Oblique attachment signal
I guess the child probably had a – I assume it's a boy – bad dream and is wanting to be comforted. * She seems really relaxed but is not responding to the child.	* Direct attachment signal
If she's not responding and feeling empathetic, you'd think either she's *resentful* of being woken up in the middle of the night or she's either *aggravated* or...	Disconnected anger
// Unless *she's trying to sort of tough love like that respond, trying to train him not to ask for attention.* Either ** *she'll break down and hug the child or calmly explain why she's not responding.* Eventually have the child agree to go back to *sleep* and she'll go back to her bedroom.	Deactivate ** fractured response Disconnect Deactivate

What is Ethan telling us here?

> I ask my attachment figure to comfort me. I'm confused! Why doesn't she respond? Is she angry with me? Why does she resent me? She is training me to not want her. Is she going to hug me? I must deactivate and shut off conscious awareness of my need for comfort so she can leave.

Ethan's story describes the intersection of behaviorism and attachment. Instead of "learning to love" (Waters et al., 1991), Ethan was taught to deactivate. Ethan and children like him remain confused about why they cannot get the comfort their biology yearns for, and they learn to shut down the expressions of their attachment needs. They learn to regulate alone. The conflict between lesson learned and what Ethan feels becomes the duality of minds and emotions. Although we can learn not to express our biological needs, we cannot exorcise them. Externally, the deactivator must appear strong and independent, but Ethan's internal confusion and longing for connection, comfort, and care remain.

Ethan's AAP stories also show his confusion about coping when anger leaks through his deactivated shell. Bowlby (1973) writes about the importance of anger in attachment relationships. Direct expressions of anger fortify relationships and contribute to attachment's protective function. Unexpressed anger violates the evolutionary function of this emotion because it can neither be acknowledged nor regulated by attachment figures. Therefore, rather than being constructive, anger becomes destructive and frightening.

Ethan demonstrates in his Bed story how worry about the mother's anger contributes to his feelings that he is not worth comfort and care, even when he asks for it. His Corner story demonstrates why he had to split off his anger. In Ethan's mind, anger serves no useful purpose. Anger is irrational and dangerous. Nothing good ever comes from it. Anger is destructive. His collapses and inability to concentrate always occurred after a breakup or an angry threat to his marriage, which now given his AAP, makes perfect sense.

One of the most profound characteristics of Failed Mourners is the paradox of how to navigate the two conflicting representational selves. It is only through Ethan's AAP stories, where he is freed from telling his own story, that we are able to see his two selves working side by side – his rational deactivation shell protecting him from his trauma. And we can see how this duality of selves and worlds works, so to speak, until it stops working. When Ethan came for assessment, his shell had stopped working and the cost of collapse and crashing had become too much to bear. He wanted to know and see what was really there, give words to that which had been silenced, and explore his past. The task of assessment and therapy was to help Ethan see and understand how failed protection was traumatic, despite his attachment figures' intentions, and how these failures had impacted his life. Only then could he feel sorrow, express and experience anger, and begin to grieve.

How to talk about Failed Mourning: A top-down or left brain approach

The representational narrative we co-create with our attachment figures is the only story we have; we hold onto it for dear life, even if it is painful (Bowlby, 1980). The AAP stories can bring a new understanding to our clients' narratives and help uncover the experiences and the defensive processes they use to create a distorted sense of safety and comfort. When talking with our clients about the AAP, we must keep in mind the vulnerability that exists around their narrative, what it holds, what it means to them, and the painful emotions that will emerge as they begin to let go of it and begin to grieve. This awareness must be balanced with the recognition that our clients are distressed when they come to us and want to discover why they feel the way they do, why something doesn't feel right. Together we co-construct a more accurate view, a shift in perspective, and a new understanding. Grief is the process of constructing a new narrative of the past in light of the present and integrating the conflicting representational selves (Bowlby, 1980, 1988).

Defensive deactivation attempts to neutralize and replace negative affect with knowledge, left brain processes (George & West, 2012). So for Ethan, and most Failed Mourners, knowledge would be the starting block to begin permeating his protective shell and help him take in the information I wanted to share with him about his attachment pattern and his AAP stories. Intellect and rational problem-solving had created a protective façade for Ethan throughout his life, and they were not going to go away overnight. My goal was not to dissolve these defenses but rather join his defensive structure and use it to help him start to logically understand that what he had been told by his attachment figures was not accurate. I wanted Ethan to become curious and inquisitive when his defensive deactivation took hold and threatened to block negative affect and painful experience. I wanted to bring answers and logical explanations to the confusion and uncertainty evidenced in his attachment stories and to the contradictory depictions he told of his parents and childhood.

When thinking about how to talk with Ethan about his testing, I also took into consideration several other factors, such as his tendency to space out, forget things, and lose focus when emotionally aroused. His neutralized attachment, which was evidenced in his descriptions of having a relatively normal childhood, his failure to describe family problems on the MMPI-2, and his remark during the Corner story of the AAP that his parents were not alcoholics or abusive, was also an important consideration, as was the fact that nothing Ethan and I were about to discuss regarding the AAP results was necessarily new information. As a clinician, I use attachment theory and research to understand my clients' struggles, dilemmas, and presenting symptoms. In the very beginning of my work with clients, I begin to describe the function of attachment, infant patterns, failed protection, attachment trauma, defensive coping, and grief. By the time Ethan and I were ready to discuss his testing, we had a solid therapeutic relationship and shared the language of attachment.

Holding all of this in mind, my left brain approach to discussing his results was to walk Ethan through each of his tests and use the data to help him see his pain and trauma. This can be a very validating experience for many clients, but especially for a Failed Mourner who has been told (and tells themselves) that there is no pain, no reason to feel sad or angry, no trauma. As Ethan and I moved through the results from his MMPI-2 and then Rorschach, the question that kept arising was *why* the testing showed so much trauma. Even though, we had already talked about the concepts of attachment trauma, failed protection, and the ways he learned to cope with distress (his deactivated shell), these discussions needed repetition. Attachment research shows how difficult it is to change our beliefs and our tendency to gravitate toward information that confirms our representational model of self and attachment figures (Sroufe et al., 2005). Our defenses distort or exclude informational misfits to fortify what we already know. The struggle for Ethan was to hold onto, believe, and integrate new information that contradicted his deactivated self. It would take repeated efforts to bring in new perspectives. The therapeutic work with Failed Mourners moves slowly, unfolding over time with the development of the relationship and ability to trust the therapist.

As we talked about the AAP, I reiterated previous conversations, stressing how he had learned to cope with his parents' ongoing dismissiveness, misattunement, and failed protection and that what he had experienced was in fact traumatic. Gradually, I reframed specific memories he had described to me as examples of failed protection that his biology would experience as attachment trauma. I talked about what happens when no one is there to help us understand and hold our emotions, how protective failures leave us feeling alone, afraid, helpless, and ashamed. I used examples from his AAP stories to highlight these emotions, as well as how he had relied on deactivation to guard against his feelings. I then introduced the concept of Failed Mourning, explaining it in a way that could help Ethan see how the deactivation coping strategies had protected him and were necessary for his survival. I also wanted him to see that these strategies came with a price. These learned strategies that had developed early in his life prevented him from being able to see what he sensed deep inside and kept him from grieving the protection he had lost. We spoke about the need for him to mourn the trauma of protective failures, just like one mourns the death of someone they love. I spoke about grieving as an innate process, and how we are biologically driven to cry and yearn and search for what we have lost. Unable to restore what we lost, we become angry and feel hopeless. Being blocked from grieving prevents us from fully living our lives (Bowlby, 1980). Ethan would have to grieve to become a whole functioning person and find the happiness he craved.

The concept of Failed Mourning resonated deeply with Ethan. By showing him the intersection between his AAP self and named experiences of trauma, he felt validated and understood. Emotional release and a relief from shame allowed him to develop hope that he could be happy and live the life he wanted. The life he deserved in face of his chronic feeling that he did not deserve to live a good life. Ethan stayed in this emotional space for a short time, long enough to get a sense of how things could be, and then his logical mind took hold (his natural deactivating defenses). He wanted a plan and asked me, "So what steps do I need to take to grieve?" I looked at him and smiled in understanding and said, "You have already begun."

Conclusion

The Failed Mourner walks into our rooms silenced; they are distressed, in pain, and unable to answer the question of why. We help them understand their emotional state from a variety of perspectives and tests during the Therapeutic Assessment process. And we answer their question of, "Why do I feel this way if there is no reason for me to feel this way?" by using their own words, images, and stories told to the AAP. The AAP is the tool that provides us with the key to unlock their inner knowing. As clinicians, we become their secure base (Bowlby, 1988). We are the wiser, kinder, stronger ones that help them name, hold, explore, and make sense of their experiences so they can grieve. We join them in their journey. To Ethan I am forever grateful that he trusted me enough to let me join him. The knowledge I have gained is far beyond any book I have ever read. Witnessing his discovery, his pain, his relief, his reconstruction, and his grief has been life changing.

Notes

1 Italics = defenses; bold = trauma; underline = agency, capacity to act
2 Italics = defenses

References

Bowlby, J. (1973). *Attachment and loss: Vol. 2. Separation: Anxiety and anger.* Basic Books.

Bowlby, J. (1980). *Attachment and loss: Vol. 3. Loss: Sadness and depression.* Basic Books.

Bowlby, J. (1982). *Attachment and loss: Vol. 1. Attachment.* Basic Books. (original publication 1969)

Bowlby, J. (1988). *A secure base.* Basic Books.

Caldwell, A. (2008, Mar. 26–27). Toward an etiological and attachment-related understanding of the origins of the MMPI-2 codetypes [Conference Presentation]. *Society for Personality Assessment 2008 Conference,* New Orleans, LA, USA.

Finn, S. (2007). *In our clients' shoes: Theory and techniques of therapeutic assessment.* Psychology Press.

Frumkin, M. R., Robinaugh, D. J., LeBlanc, N. J., Ahmad, Z., Bui, E., Nock, M. K., Simon, N. M., & McNally, R. J. (2021). The pain of grief: Exploring the concept of psychological pain and its relation to complicated grief, depression, and risk for suicide in bereaved adults. *Journal of Clinical Psychology,* 77(1), 254–267. https://doi.org/10.1002/jclp.23024

George, C., & Solomon, J. (2008). The caregiving system: A behavioral systems approach to parenting. In J. Cassidy & P. R. Shaver (Eds.), *Handbook of attachment: Theory, research, and clinical applications* (2nd ed., pp. 833–856). Guilford Press.

George, C., & West, M. (2012). *The adult attachment projective picture system: Attachment theory and assessment in adults.* Guilford Press.

Hesse, E. (2016). The adult attachment interview: Protocol, method of analysis, and selected empirical studies: 1985–2015. In J. Cassidy & P. Shaver (Eds.), *Handbook of attachment: Theory, research, and clinical applications* (pp. 553–597). Guilford Press.

Kamphuis, J. H., Kugeares, S. L., & Finn, S. E. (2000). Rorschach correlates of sexual abuse: Trauma content and aggression indexes. *Journal of Personality Assessment,* 75(2), 212–224. https://doi.org/10.1207/S15327752JPA7502_3

Parkes, C. M. (2006). *Love and loss.* Routledge.

Perry, B. D., Pollard, R. A., Blakley, T. L., Baker, W. L., & Vigilante, D. (1995). Childhood trauma, the neurobiology of adaptation, and "use dependent" development of the brain: How "states" become "traits." *Infant Mental Health Journal,* 16(4), 271–289. https://doi.org/10.1002/1097-0355(199524)16:4<271::AID-IMHJ2280160404>3.0.CO;2-B

Simon and Garfunkel, Simon, P., & Scoppa, B. (2001). *Sounds of silence.*

Solomon, J., & George, C. (1996). Defining the caregiving system: Toward a theory of caregiving. *Infant Mental Health Journal,* 17(3), 183–197. https://doi.org/0.1002/(SICI)1097-0355(199623)17:3<198::AID-IMHJ2>3.0.CO;2-L

Solomon, J., George, C., & De Jong, A. (1995). Children classified as controlling at age six: Evidence of disorganized representational strategies and aggression at home and at school. *Development and Psychopathology,* 7(3), 447–463. https://doi.org/10.1017/S0954579400006623

Sroufe, L. A., Egeland, B., Carlson, E. A., & Collins, A. W. (2005). *The development of the person.* Guilford Press.

Van Der Kolk, B. A. (2006). Clinical implications of neuroscience research in PTSD. *Annals of the New York Academy of Sciences,* 1071(1), 277–293. https://doi.org/10.1196/annals.1364.022

6 Opening the attachment trauma floodgates

Preoccupation with Personal Suffering

Caroline Lee and Carol George

Preoccupation with Personal Suffering is a form of incomplete mourning that Bowlby (1980) termed pathological mourning. The inability to complete the mourning process is an assault on mental health. Preoccupied with Personal Suffering produces a state of mind analogous to post-traumatic stress where clients are confused about experiences of childhood trauma and unable to differentiate between threat and safety. The result is a view of the world and relationships as perpetually threatening; clients live in an entangled web of frightening attachment trauma. The primary defensive posture of this state of mind is cognitive disconnection, the primary regulatory defense of individuals with preoccupied attachment status (see Chapter 1). The defensive exclusion goal is to split (literally disconnect) experience and affect (Bowlby, 1980), which creates a mental fog that blurs conscious access to biographical memory. As a result, clients become confused about what they believe they experienced and what their parents told them was "true." This contradictory set of competing representational models becomes a tremendous source of mental confusion and pain when trauma is involved. Frightening affect is, therefore, either ever-present, dictating every move, experience, and relationship, or affect is blurred and diluted so that the only recognizable residue of trauma is unexplained feelings of anxiety and terror (see Chapter 4). This chapter uses a case illustration to demonstrate how the Adult Attachment Projective Picture System (AAP) brings light to Preoccupied with Personal Suffering and the disconnected models of the traumatized client living in an emotional "war zone" (George & West, 2012).

The case of Catherine

Catherine, a 36-year-old African-American female, initially sought individual therapy from the first author in 2018. At the time, she was living with her parents while on leave from her job as an evangelical missionary to college students. Catherine had grown weary of her mission work and sought therapy to discover why she felt so lost and considered other avenues for work. Living at home was difficult, and she began talking about how anxious she was staying with her parents. She had lived away

DOI: 10.4324/9781003215431-8

from her parents for almost 20 years, attending college then becoming a missionary, which often led to missionary assignments overseas. Now at home, she noticed how uncomfortable she felt around her father, noting she had forgotten how intense he was and how his volatility required people to walk on eggshells.

Catherine spoke of her family's background as therapy continued. Her parents immigrated from West Africa in their twenties so her father could attend medical school. They had two children shortly after that, Catherine being the youngest. Her mother stayed home with Catherine and her older brother while her father attended medical school. Her father abruptly returned to West Africa when Catherine was six. She could not recall knowing why he left or when he would return. He returned as suddenly as he left when she was 12.

Catherine was curious why she had few childhood memories and was confused about her discomfort with her father. When asked about her relationship with her parents, her narrative wandered and was confusing and contradictory.

> My parents were good and made sure we had everything we needed. My father was a little angry at times. Yeah. I guess but I don't know, they took care of me and my brother. I wish my mom could have paid attention to me more, but my brother struggled and was angry all the time. She had to take care of him, and I was okay. So yeah, mostly things were good, I guess.

Unfortunately, therapy was cut short after only a few sessions when Catherine was assigned to a new mission that required a long-distance move. Her anxiety about her family began to dissipate as she settled into her new assignment. Her life was highly structured and busy with missionary responsibilities: weekly discipleship groups, bible studies, fundraising meetings, church events, and one-on-one engagements with college students. She did not pursue additional therapy, but instead met with her church mentor for support. As their relationship grew, she told her mentor about her relentless anxiety, sadness, and numbness. She felt shut down and empty inside even though she could follow through with her weekly commitments. Catherine also discussed with her mentor how she wanted to find a partner and have children but was confused about why she was terrified to date. She wanted to become more comfortable around men.

Around this time, Catherine developed romantic feelings toward a staff member on her missionary team. Rather than pursuing the relationship, she was afraid and started avoiding in-person contact altogether. Nevertheless, she longed to be close to him and found herself taking walks by his condo, hoping to run into him. Curious about Catherine's conflict, her mentor began asking questions about her relationship with

her father. She said she had few memories of her father, which she explained was because of his six-year hiatus from the family in middle
childhood. As Catherine's desire to be with her teammate grew, she
started feeling out of control and did not trust her feelings, believing
they were sinful. She also started having nightmares and sudden "frightening blurry memories" from her childhood, which led her to seek more
support from her mentor. For the first time, these memories were disturbing. She remembered her father openly watching and showing her
pornography in her childhood home and vague nightmares of her father
sneaking into her room at night. Her mentor now suggested she find a
therapist.

Two years after ending a brief therapy with the first author, Catherine
reached out to inquire about additional treatment. The possibility of a
Therapeutic Assessment had been introduced during her prior treatment
because she had questions about her anxiety and ambivalence toward
her missionary work. Now, her questions were about trauma. She won-
dered if her memories were real or was she crazy and "coming off the
rails." The only assessment possibility because of her living situation was
telehealth. She agreed that a telehealth Therapeutic Assessment seemed
to be the best path at this time. The first author and Catherine spent
the first sessions developing questions for the assessment. Her questions
were: Why don't I trust men? How has my relationship with my parents
affected me? Why do I shut down so easily? Why am I sad all of the time?
Have I experienced trauma? Could my memories be real?

Catherine's "shut down" response was evident as she struggled to articulate her thoughts in the session. She quickly became derailed and
confused, as if she was becoming consciously aware of her disparate understanding of self and her childhood. Although Catherine was terrified,
she preferred to view herself as crazy rather than consider the possibility
that she was abused as a child.

> I'm having dreams of my father sneaking into my room at night and
> I wake up screaming STOP! I'm pretty sure though it's just a dream.
> But I also have images of sitting with my dad while he watched por-
> nography. But everything is blurry, and it makes no sense that would
> have actually happened to me. I feel like I'm really just coming off
> the rails, and something is wrong with me.

Catherine noted that her frightening memories and nightmares increased
as interest in dating her colleague grew. This clearly confused her, unable to assimilate that her feelings of failed protection were activated.
She had managed to disconnect and blur out these painful memories for
the majority of her life. The initial assessment session made clear that
Catherine's attachment history was a list of lifetime assaults, as summarized in Table 6.1.

Table 6.1 Catherine's Attachment Trauma

Developmental Trauma	Precipitating Attachment Events
Father unpredictably enraged	Attachment system activated by
Father abandoned family, age 6–12	close relationship with mentor
Passive/neglectful mother	→ Conscious realization of
Racial and cultural trauma	attachment needs
Blurry Memories:	
Inundated with porn by father	Fear of men and sexuality
Unclear if sexually abused by father	Shame of sexual feelings

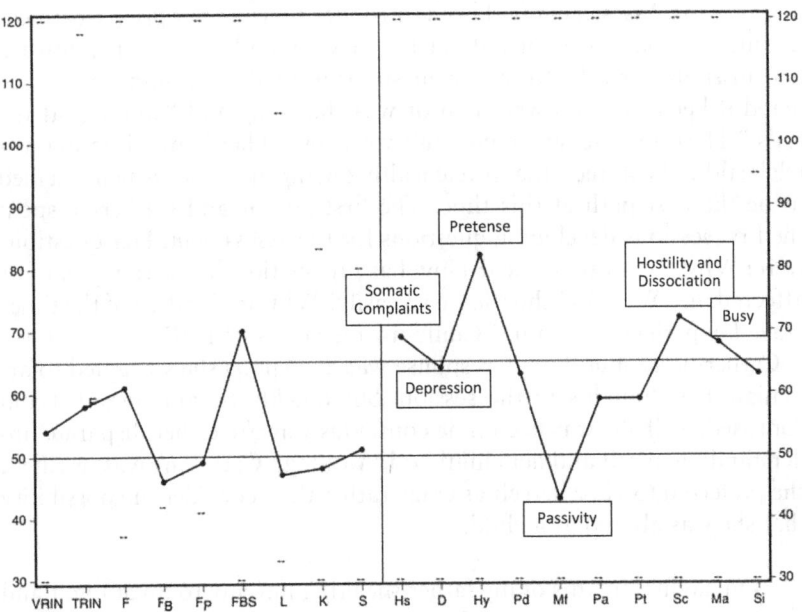

Figure 6.1 Catherine's MMPI.

Test results

Catherine engaged in a Brief Therapeutic Assessment (Finn, 2007). Two assessments were used to help address her questions. One was the Minnesota Multiphasic Personality Inventory-Second Edition (MMPI-2). The other was the AAP.

The results of Catherine's MMPI are shown in Figure 6.1.

The MMPI-2 results highlight her affective "war zone" and some of the underlying reasons for her other complaints, including increasing chronic stomach pain, sadness, dissociation, and paralyzing passivity in her relationships. These results also show Catherine's attempts to contain (i.e., regulate) her traumatic distress: pretense (referred to as denial on the MMPI-2) and keeping busy. The MMPI-2 results provide a glimpse of what will be fully elucidated in the AAP described in the next section as cognitive disconnection exclusion strategies.

During the extended inquiry, Catherine's response to the results suggesting underlying depression was confusing and contradictory. Her first response was surprise, as if she was not aware of having depressed affect. The discussion moved to dissociation, which was connected to her assessment question about shutting down. She shared, "Sometimes I am mid-conversation, and my brain just turns off. It is difficult to keep speaking, and I don't understand why that keeps happening to me!" One explanation was she possibly dissociates from her feelings to prevent overwhelm. Dissociation can feel like cognitively shutting down, suddenly unable to think clearly. She agreed with this interpretation and spoke about how she dissociates more when around her family. When asked about her parents' response to sadness, she shared her parents would have punished her if she had expressed sadness in their presence. She recalled that they emphasized being happy and polite to "fit in" her predominantly White school and neighborhood. Could dissociation be protecting her from underlying sadness? Might her brain "turn off" when she comes close to her sad feelings? Catherine left the session with a deeper understanding of her distress, amazed at how "bad" she had been feeling. Still, she smiled while speaking about her sadness. The hope was that the AAP would provide more insight into the adaptive origins of her problems and address her questions about trauma and her relationships with her parents.

Catherine's AAP

We began this chapter by describing what it means to be Preoccupied with Personal Suffering. Here, we provide the reader with selections of Catherine's most characteristic stories that evidence her state of mind. These stories demonstrate how cognitive disconnection defensively blurs Catherine's conscious traumatic realization. The stories evidence traumatic segregated systems and derealization that indicate a distorted representational flight from attachment reality (see Chapter 4).

Catherine's alone stories illustrate painful disconnected contradictory models of her attachment self and experience. Bowlby (1980) proposed that parents enforce their model of events and the parent-child relationship as the child's predominant memory. The parent's model subordinates the child's model, which develops when the child knows they had a qualitatively different experience than the parents' rendition of their reality. Defensive exclusion processes disconnect the two sets of models but fail to completely "squash" (i.e., repress) the child's view of the parent and self. As such, the child's experience sneaks into consciousness. The child faces the dilemma of deciding what is real. Which "story" is true? Fearing rejection and abandonment, survival depends on endorsing the parent's view of the relationship. However, the child continues to be plagued by diffuse feelings of unease because the disconnection is incomplete (Bowlby, 1980).

Catherine's parents enforced the following representational model, "I make promises to be together, I come, and we do things together." Catherine's corresponding self-model is "I wait for you. I hope you come." But her model of her real parent is "You don't keep promises. You betray me time after time." And her self-model is I'm shocked. I can't tell you how angry and guilty I feel. Your betrayal sends my mind spinning. You feel dead to me. I must harden my heart against your betrayal and pretend we are happy so we can go forward.

Here is Catherine's response to Window[1]:

She *waits* for her dad to come home. He is not coming,	Disconnect
but *she doesn't know that*. She *waits and waits*. Maybe	Disconnect
he *promised to do something but just didn't keep his*	Trauma – betrayal
word. She is *hopeful*, but she is also *shocked*. She's	Disconnect,
in *disbelief*, like *trying to believe*. He said he would	Trauma, Dereal
come, but he's not here. *She is let down, let down in*	
her heart. She still looks for him when he promises	Trauma – betrayal
things, but she grows up being let down, so yeah. She	
just *cuts him off. I mean she's cordial, still there, but*	Disconnect
in her heart, she definitely cut him off. She has learned	
not to expect much.	

Catherine's Window story describes her experience of and response to her father's betrayal. She starts with disconnection, hoping yet knowing in her heart that her father will break his promise. When she realizes the truth of her reality, she becomes shocked, which according to Bowlby (1980), is a person's initial response to loss. The story shows how Catherine's disbelief becomes a surreal attempt to understand and integrate these disparate, contradictory models of being, furthering our understanding of Catherine's experiences of dissociation. "Did this happen to me? Could my memories be real?" Dissociation represents her attempted flight from reality that, although her father promised her he would come, he abandoned her. Catherine manages the pain of this "lost" attachment figure by describing a disconnected self. She tells how the story character engages in a charade to preserve the real-world relationship with her father but underlying her "cordial" exterior is a hardened heart full of pain, disappointment, and grief. According to Bowlby (1973), this state of mind is preferable to realizing the terror of feeling abandoned and alone.

Here is Catherine's Bench story[2]:

I don't know what led up to the scene. But um, I	Disconnect
think that this person will *spend a very long time*	Disconnected shame
trying to cover up that this is how they feel all the	
time, a lot. I think they feel *alone* and **abandoned,**	Trauma
um yeah, and **shocked** and **disbelief.** ...There are	Trauma
people there **but no one there that could um really**	Derealization
um connect and comfort this individual. They	Trauma
just *try and put on a face like nothing happened,* I	Disconnect
think in their own way, maybe try and communicate	
like I'm not ok, but *when that gets missed, they*	Disconnect
just learn to not even do that much. They might	
manipulate to get other people to feel for them.	Disconnect

Catherine unveils the fears she implied in her Window story. The projected self (person) is alone and abandoned, described now with a sense of desperation (no one that could comfort this individual). She is not physically alone; however, she has to pretend to be okay because the people who are present (presumably attachment figures) would not see her distress in any case. Catherine portrays the character with the typical passivity that develops in preoccupied attachment and ambivalent-resistant children (Marvin et al., 2016). The self passively signals for help by "maybe trying to communicate I'm not ok" which doesn't get noticed. She has a second attempt to signal, which takes the form of feisty "look at me" manipulative behavior (Marvin et al., 2016), as suggested by Catherine's story ending.

The AAP dyadic stimuli portray individuals in potential attachment relationships. Catherine's dyadic stories also reveal contradictory attachment models of self and attachment figure. The parent's dominant model of their relationship, "I take care of you. Everything is okay," enforces Catherine to endorse a representation of trust, "I will wait because I trust you." Catherine's subordinate model is, "I am angry, in pain, and feeling abandoned. I can only cope if I withhold my distress and pretend to be okay." She knows in her heart that the parent's model is a charade, "Your expressions of closeness are a sham. Your betrayal sends my mind spinning and you feel dead to me."

Here is Catherine's Bed story:

It looks like the child is definitely reaching out to their	*Attachment signal,
mother * but it's *unclear if the mother is reaching*	disconnect
back out or if her hand is clasped. It just seems	
like the child is reaching way more for the mother,	
like there is closeness there * but the mother is not	*Attachment signal
reaching back in the same way. It doesn't seem as kind	
of open. The child probably maybe had a *hard day or*	Heightened
just in general, just you know, wants affection and	attachment need
attention. The mother has a lot on her mind trying to	Disconnected
	caregiver

make it loves her child, but she just has a lot going on.
She isn't even aware of her child's emotional needs.
The child is still pretty innocent is *still wants attention*   Heightened
and affection, and um, you know, will eventually   attachment need
come to the conclusion that they are not going to get
that. The mom eventually wants to, yeah, just wants
to be there.

This story reveals the conundrum of the ambivalent child. Catherine repeats her heightened attachment need throughout the story. She refers twice to reaching, an attachment signal for physical contact, and after some hesitation suggests that there does not even need to be a reason to want affection. The conundrum is Catherine trying to make sense of why the mother would be there in the first place and not respond. She describes the mother as distracted, and like her dissolving hope for the father to come home in Window, comes to understand that her mother will not notice and give her what she wants. At the end of the story, the mother is just there. The mother does not acknowledge the child. The mother does not pretend to be sensitive; she never responds to the child's attachment signal. The Bed story shows the "swirl" of Catherine's disconnected representational models as she shifts back and forth between the dominant model (We're close and love each other) and the subordinate model (You don't notice me or take care of me) – "the child is reaching way more for the mother, like there is closeness there but the mother is not reaching back."

After the AAP administration, Catherine was asked about the personal relevance of this story. Catherine told more about the effects of her father's absence in middle childhood.

> My mom was just trying to make it while my dad was away. She was kind of absent. There was closeness at times, but I always wanted her to be more involved in my life. I just tried not to make things harder for her. She had a lot going on taking care of my brother.

Cognitive disconnection helps Catherine name but not "know" about her attachment losses and how they have affected her sense of self and attachment relationships. Adopting her mother's model allows Catherine to stay emotionally close enough to her mother to regulate fear, concluding, "My mother is functionally present, so I am safe."

Catherine's attachment pattern is Preoccupied with Personal Suffering. Her attachment figures were neither sensitive nor protective. At best, they were functionally present, and at worst, they were hostile and betrayed and abandoned her. Catherine's stories lack agency of self, as is common with Preoccupied individuals. She shows no capacity to act to manage her attachment distress, and she cannot think (internalized secure base) about attachment because she is so disconnected and confused. Catherine found a way to go forward by adopting her parents' dominant relationship model and pretending that everything was okay. To do this, Catherine had to blur her real experiences and feelings (i.e., disconnect), often dissociating from the shock and pain of betrayal and abandonment. Her war zone is haunted by unconscious shame and self-reproach and the inability to understand why she feels the way she does.

Therapeutic Assessment

After completing the AAP, the assessor (first author) had a new understanding of what Catherine had endured. The AAP allowed Catherine to see her attachment trauma in the form of stories about hypothetical people, validating her blurry memories of her caregivers' unavailability, abandonment, and betrayal – her attachment trauma. Catherine and the assessor returned to her AAP stories in a later session, and with support Catherine was able to describe the shock and betrayal she felt remembering her father showing her pornography and sneaking into her room at night. Her memories became more explicit as she began trusting and understanding her assessment results.

Preoccupied with Personal Suffering is a form of chronic incomplete mourning (Bowlby, 1980). Catherine began to move in the direction of completing the mourning process by naming and understanding her attachment losses. The Therapeutic Assessment with the AAP helped her see she needed more support to repair her fractured self. In the role of the assessor, the first author wrote her a Therapeutic Assessment letter summarizing the results and suggested she find a therapist in her city of residence to help her mourn and repair. Here are excerpts of her letter:

> Catherine, your AAP stories suggested that you had experiences as a child that left you feeling isolated, abandoned, shocked, and helpless, and suggested you grew up constantly frightened. This has been confusing and hard to understand because you were told that there was no reason to feel the way you do. You brilliantly figured out how to keep moving forward with your life by pretending you were okay and staying disconnected from yourself and your family.
>
> Recent scary memories have overwhelmed you. You have worked hard to understand what really happened to you as a child. We learned together that your parents did not protect you. Psychologists call this "attachment trauma." The good news, Catherine, is that people can heal from attachment trauma by building a secure and safe relationship with a therapist. You've already begun to grieve the losses you endured as a child and are working hard to heal from the chronic suffering you have survived since childhood. You need continued support to heal from the lack of protection and the pain you have carried all these years.

Often, clients enter the therapy room searching for answers about why they think, feel, and behave in certain ways in their current life. They are filled with shame about how they interact with others and engage in the world because they lack a clear understanding of how their early interactions with caregivers affected them. Catherine's question, "Why do I shut down so easily?" is a perfect example of such a phenomenon and illuminates how she is in search of a "new" reason for her behavior besides her "old" self-blaming explanation of "I am crazy." The AAP can help clients understand the "why" – why they behave in certain ways and that they are not at fault; they instead had no choice. They had to find some way, some solution to survive the emotional pain and overwhelm from their childhoods. This kind of understanding can help reduce the shame clients feel, which then opens the door for grieving what one had to endure and the effects it has had on their life. Here is another excerpt from Catherine's letter addressing her question: "Why do I shut down so easily?"

> Catherine, you necessarily shut down after being attacked and frightened by your father. You shared painful childhood memories of your father going "ballistic" and were afraid he would kill himself if you responded with anger. Shutting down keeps your anger at bay and protects you from being abandoned or further attacked. Your parents also made you feel guilty when you shared your longings and needs. You learned to stay safe by shutting down and pretending you were ok. Your testing results showed you experience dissociation, which is a form of shutting down. Dissociation prevents us from getting emotionally overwhelmed but can often leave us feeling numb and shut down as a result. You had no choice but to dissociate and now need support to learn new ways of coping when you are afraid.

Treatment goal

The goal of treatment for preoccupied sufferers is repair and integration. They have survived by disconnecting attachment experience and affect into two representational models. The AAP uncovered these models and showed that, although contradictory, they were coherent. Her parent model required her to pretend to stay connected; her self-model represented the painful truth of failed protection during her childhood. Preoccupied sufferers need help naming failed protection and grieving the lost attachment relationship, especially the lost self. Grieving helps individuals feel the truth of their failed protection and clearly see the path of integration: "You did not protect me. It was not my fault. I am worthy of care" George and Solomon (2008).

With support, Catherine also needed to feel the sorrow of knowing that a real reunion with and protection from her lost attachment figures was not possible given their current state of mind. The final step of the Therapeutic Assessment was to help Catherine continue on her path of discovery by finding a local psychotherapist to support her in the process of mourning and reuniting with her core attachment self.

Notes

1 Italics = defenses; bold = trauma
2 Italics = defenses; bold = trauma

References

Bowlby, J. (1973). *Attachment and loss: Vol. 2. Separation: Anxiety and anger.* Basic Books.

Bowlby, J. (1980). *Attachment and loss: Vol. 3. Loss: Sadness and depression.* Basic Books.

Finn, S. (2007). *In our clients' shoes: Theory and techniques of therapeutic assessment.* Psychology Press.

George, C., & West, M. (2012). *The adult attachment projective picture system: Attachment theory and assessment in adults.* Guilford Press.

Main, M., & Hesse, E. (1990). Parents' unresolved traumatic experiences are related to infant disorganized attachment status: Is frightened and/or frightening parental behavior the linking mechanism? In M. T. Greenberg, D. Cicchetti, & E. M. Cummings (Eds.), *Attachment in the preschool years* (pp. 161–182). University of Chicago Press.

Marvin, R. S., Britner, P. A., & Russell, B. S. (2016). Normative development: The ontogeny of childhood attachment. In J. Cassidy & P. R. Shaver (Eds.), *Handbook of attachment: Theory, research, and clinical applications* (3rd ed., pp. 273–290). Guilford Press.

Solomon, J., & George, C. (2021). The attachment antecedents of shame. *Attachment: New Directions in Psychotherapy and Relational Psychoanalysis, 15*(2), 159–180. https://doi.org/10.33212/att.v15n2.2021.159

7 Pain, misery, and suffering

Unresolved attachment as a predictor of treatment outcome in male combat-related Post-Traumatic Stress Disorder

Deane E. Aikins and Julie Wargo Aikins

Welcome to Recon country. Pain, misery, and suffering await you here.
– *Amphibious Reconnaissance Marine Corps Poster*

After 20 years of war, what is the status of available treatments for combat Post-Traumatic Stress Disorder (PTSD)? There are no empirically supported therapy algorithms for the treatment of PTSD. Conceptualized from a "one-size-fits-all" perspective, the Veteran must navigate among alternatives, including two FDA-approved medications, several evidence-based treatments (EBTs), or other treatment modalities with less empirical support or qualified provider availability. Unfortunately, despite well-established and documented treatment benefits in civilian populations, these offerings are noted to have a sizeable premature termination rate and smaller effect sizes for military populations (Litz et al., 2019; Steenkamp et al., 2020). For these reasons, it seems imperative to reform how we think about and treat combat Veterans diagnosed with PTSD. We suggest that shifting the view from a "one-size-fits-all" perspective to a more individualized approach may be beneficial. This type of personalized care would consider differences in attachment, emotion regulation, and interpersonal relatedness – all essential facets of one's mental and emotional well-being that have been overlooked in the current treatment milieu. As such, we believe that differences in attachment status, namely incomplete pathological mourning for trauma, could partially account for and likely predict the diminished effects found in EBTs with military populations. In this chapter, we discuss the case of a treatment-seeking, 30-year-old African-American male who is a combat Veteran of Operation Enduring Freedom in Afghanistan as an exemplar of how knowing his Unresolved attachment classification helps interpret observed difficulties with the standard Veterans Administration (VA) treatment program. His attachment status is considered in addition to a panel of empirically validated measures of PTSD symptomatology, emotion dysregulation, and personality. Finally, the value of using the *Adult Attachment Projective Picture System* (AAP) to guide personalized

DOI: 10.4324/9781003215431-9

treatment for Veterans with similar profiles as our case study will be considered as a research-driven therapeutic alternative for patients.

Historical background

Childhood history

Mr. Evans is a 30-year-old African American male born in a Midwestern city. He reported that his biological mother had substance abuse problems and abandoned him before age 1. Mr. Evans was raised by his father, who had a history of significant alcohol use. He stated being close to his father as a child and in adulthood, "I love my dad- I have the best dad on the planet. I would die for him. He's the shit." Mr. Evans reported having his father's name tattooed on his right shoulder because "he always used to carry me around in his right arm, and now I carry him around on mine." Mr. Evans has several half-siblings, all from different fathers. These half-siblings were first in foster care and then put up for adoption, "we grew up separately, so for the most part, I was an only child." Mr. Evans witnessed several traumatic experiences early on, including exposure to gun violence at age 10 and seeing a dead body when he was 11. He was frequently left alone, staying by himself after school since second grade as his father worked late hours. Mr. Evans started drinking alcohol at the age of two, when his father and family members would give it to him on special occasions, such as holidays or weddings.

Military history

After high school, Mr. Evans tried several college courses and training programs without completion. Eventually, he joined the Marine Corps "to make something" of himself as an Infantryman. He wanted to succeed in the Marine Corps, intending to become an Amphibious Reconnaissance Marine, an elite level of Marines who serve as the Special Forces of the Corps. Mr. Evans deployed to a region of Afghanistan that was characterized by high levels of combat. He experienced multiple trauma exposures of combat-related injury and death during his deployment.

Mr. Evans' primary adult trauma stemmed from a day when he was placed on radio duty while his unit was sent on vehicle patrol. A teammate was killed by enemy fire while sitting in a position that Mr. Evans usually held. He said, "that was my bullet, my buddy was killed –shot in the head, and it should have been my bullet." Following the loss of his teammate, he related that he no longer wanted to "try hard for anything" and began to drink heavily. He reflected that his drinking ended his brief marriage. Following his divorce, he had a DUI and was injured when that vehicle crashed.

Veteran history

After his military service, Mr. Evans began to experience a downward spiral of distress, poor functioning, and adverse life events that included several years of court proceedings, with significant ramifications. After his honorable discharge from the Marine Corps, he was arrested following a bar fight and served a month in jail. Soon after his release, he was arrested again for felony firearm possession. During this period of his life, Mr. Evans engaged with the VA to receive services that provided him housing subsidies, employment placement, and legal aid.

Mr. Evans also experienced stressful interpersonal events. As an initial solution to finding housing after his jail time, he served as the caretaker of his estranged mother, who became terminally ill. He also had his first child following a brief relationship with a woman with schizophrenia. Critically, he also became highly avoidant of interpersonal interactions. This situation had significant consequences for his ability to provide for his family. He could only tolerate night shifts in janitorial work, which led to increasing court problems as he began missing hearings and sobriety tests. Mr. Evans became homeless and struggled to pay child support. He began a new relationship with the mother of his second child. Together, they raised his two daughters and five children from her previous relationships.

Mr. Evans' maladaptive coping strategies became more evident in response to these stressful life events. At this time, Mr. Evans' alcohol consumption increased to the point where the court mandated substance treatment. His inability to successfully manage his conflicting work and treatment schedules caused the court to threaten him with jail time. Mr. Evans' first hospitalization followed a suicide attempt in which he contacted the VA Suicide Hotline while intoxicated. Whereas time in the inpatient program gave him the structure necessary to begin the early phases of sobriety, PTSD symptoms of nightmares, anger, and distress around groups of people increased after his successful discharge. Unfortunately, his mother passed away close to Memorial Day. That loss, combined with the significance of the holiday, destabilized Mr. Evans's court appearances and placed his alcohol rehabilitation in jeopardy. As his instability escalated, Mr. Evans placed a second call to the Suicide Hotline. As a result, the court required Mr. Evans to complete a VA PTSD treatment program.

Assessment

At the beginning of his PTSD treatment, Mr. Evans was offered the opportunity to participate in our ongoing VA research protocol. That research aimed to use the AAP in conjunction with other measures of emotion regulation and personality to predict treatment outcomes with VA PTSD providers. All Veterans enrolling in PTSD treatment are provided an opportunity to participate in our research assessment session that occurs after the hospital standard introductory diagnostic interview but prior to the start of treatment. As such, Mr. Evans was not told of his attachment classification status, but this case is illustrative of how Veterans who fit his profile may likely share his difficulties engaging effectively in treatment.

From the assessment session, Mr. Evans' scores on the Beck Depression Inventory (BDI; Beck et a., 1996) and PTSD Checklist (PCL-V; Weathers et al., 2013) were in the range of what is typically considered severe and clinically indicated for treatment. His Difficulties with Emotion Regulation Scale (DERS; Gratz & Roemer, 2004) results indicated he had problems with his awareness and understanding of emotions, acceptance of emotions, ability to control impulses, and follow goals in the presence of negative affect. He also showed problems with access to emotion regulation strategies that are perceived to be effective for feeling better. Mr. Evans was also identified as having an overall interpersonal style described as Cold/Distant and Passive as per the Inventory of Interpersonal Problems-32 (IIP-32; Horowitz et al., 1988).

Adult Attachment Projective Picture System

Mr. Evans's overall AAP attachment classification was Unresolved chronic mourning. This classification was expectable given Mr. Evans' history of childhood attachment trauma, military trauma, and trauma during his Veteran years. Unresolved attachment is characterized by defenses that fail to contain representational traumatic attachment material that has been segregated as a means for sequestering these thoughts and experiences (see Chapter 1). Resultantly the individual experiences dysregulation that makes them feel out of control and overwhelmed.

Alone stories

The AAP uses stimuli that depict the main character(s) as alone or in dyadic relationships to understand an individual's ability to use social relationships and internalized representations to support their attachment needs. The alone pictures assess an individual's ability to either tell a story that accesses their secure internal representations or one in which they can seek attachment safety when needed. When individuals are unable to tell stories that encompass these elements, the hope is that they can act in ways that create change or take care of the issues at hand. Either integrated agency or capacity to act is necessary to reinstate regulation and resolve feelings and behaviors disorganized by fear, helplessness, and isolation (see Chapter 1).

Mr. Evans' alone stories reflect his dysregulated attachment. In both stories presented below, Mr. Evans tells stories that revolve around themes of traumatic fear, pain, and isolation. The protagonist (projected self) in Bench needs help. However, he can neither receive it from others nor act in a manner that allows him to achieve it independently, leading to the overall Unresolved classification. In the Corner story, Mr. Evans depicts the self as a little boy who is tremendously frightened in response to a punishment he is receiving for doing something wrong. The attachment dysregulation is contained (i.e., regulated) by his attempts to protect himself. However, the little boy continues to be afraid and notably feels hurt before he even gets hit. Mr. Evans tries to smooth over the situation by "wishing him the best." Deactivation is used as a regulated defensive process. Here is Mr. Evans' Bench story[1]:

I see me in this picture. I feel like I've been there.	Commentary
They need help. They in *pain*. Might be *locked up*. I see	Trauma
brick walls and this bench. It's very familiar scene. It's	Trauma
something she did that put 'em in this position or somebody	Disconnect
did something to them. They feel sad or hurt, *pain... pain*.	Trauma

And here is Mr. Evans' Corner story[2]:

That's a little boy he did something *wrong, maybe*	Deactivate
he's being punished for it. He's uh trying to protect itself	Agency:
trying to defend itself against something that's coming at	action
him, he's uh, his *back is against the wall*, it must be coming	Trauma
towards his face, his hands are out and up. Whatever is in	
front of him he don't want nothing to do with it, and he's	
thinking "I hope I don't get *hit* or ...no... stop... don't... ." I	Trauma
think he's feeling *afraid*, I think that he's feeling *fearful*. He's	Trauma
already *hurt* 'fore he get *hit*. Hopefully just get his *whoopin'*	Trauma
and keep it moving. Whatever happen, I wish him the best.	

Mr. Evans began the Bench story with a personal commentary, a remark that lets the reader know that this story is about him. This statement demonstrates the degree to which he could relate to trauma he "saw" in these AAP scenes. He described the trauma of the projected self in Bench as endangered (pain) and isolated (locked up, walls). The scene depicted in the Corner story, the last in the AAP sequence, is often highly provocative for traumatized individuals. Mr. Evans' negative view of self is the first thought that comes to mind, and knowing what is coming later in the story, he seizes on the agency to protect himself. The "meat" of the story is traumatic abuse, describing in even more detail than in Bench images of the endangered, frightened, and isolated self.

Dyadic stories

The AAP dyadic pictures portray characters in adult-adult or adult-child pairs proximal to one another. Each pair depicts a potential attachment figure who can provide comfort, sensitive and responsive caregiving, or allay feelings of danger, fear, and helplessness.

The Bed and Ambulance stories are presented below to illustrate that Mr. Evans' attachment dysregulation is also observable in his dyadic stories. Here, Mr. Evans also uses deactivation as an organized regulating strategy. In the Bed story, the limited reciprocity between the mother and child is notable; she offers him a hug, but this is not in response to an attachment bid or need. Mr. Evans suggests love between the mother and son, but there is a limited indication that he truly understands what love is. Instead, the story seems rote and routine, sounding more like a bedtime script. In the Ambulance story, Mr. Evans again uses deactivation, including authority figures and images, to contain dysregulation. Mr. Evans' real-life experiences were with an abandoning mother and an inconsistently available father. Here, he tells a story of loss and pain. A nurse or unidentified family member functionally contains the situation by explaining it will "be alright" yet consistent with the other stories, there is no warmth or sensitive caregiving. Here is Mr. Evans' Bed story[3]:

A mother and son and it's bedtime. He don't wanna go. So he getting a hug before he gets tucked in and he's thinking "I love you mommy" and she's thinking "I love you too." Love. Next, he might get a *story*, he might fall *asleep*, she might leave the room and cut out the lights. It's bedtime. I think they feeling love. He's tired and *sleepy*, and she probably is too.	Deactivate Deactivate Deactivate

And here is his Ambulance story[4]:

There's an ambulance and they're carrying someone and a *coroner*. Somebody young just *lost* protection somebody dear to them. A *nurse or a family* **member** is trying to explain to this child that everything's gonna be alright. If that's his only parent, he gonna be put in the system, unless he's got some relatives to take care of him. Lot of grieving gonna be happening. She'll probably *be instrumental in what happens next*. He's *confused*. Hurt. *Pain* ...thinkin: "it's not real, this isn't really happening... what am I gonna do? *Lost*.	Deactivate trauma Disconnect, functional synchrony Deactivate Disconnect, trauma Trauma

Across both alone and dyadic stories, Mr. Evans reveals traumatic material in stories that communicate the degree of pain and fear he feels. In Ambulance, he is also forthright in telling us about how confused he is about his trauma and who his caregivers might be. He was able to contain his dysregulation when he could "see" a potential caregiver in Ambulance but is essentially left helpless and frightened when he had to face trauma alone in Bench. Mr. Evans' challenging childhood environment conveyed real risks that exacerbated the images of danger and parental failed protection portrayed in his stories (George & Solomon, 2008). Mr. Evans likely internalized a working model of others as being unable to be safe and of self as not being worthy of protection. When environmental dangers were present as a child, his mother was absent, and his father was mainly unavailable to assuage his distress. Neither Mr. Evans' mother nor father served as a haven of safety during his childhood. Mr. Evans idealizes his father because he needs to believe there was one attachment figure willing to provide care. All evidence suggests that his father was primarily absent or endangering as well (e.g., leaving him home alone while he worked, providing him with alcohol at a young age), thereby leaving Mr. Evans isolated and needing to fend for himself. Traumatic events within Mr. Evans's childhood experiences (e.g., neighborhood violence and exposure to death), while difficult to manage regardless, might have been tolerable or easier to handle in the context of available parents. However, in a setting where parents are absent, and already beyond their limits, Mr. Evans' social, emotional, and psychological development was significantly impaired (Garbarino et al., 1991). Thoughts and feelings about his parent-child relationships appear to confuse Mr. Evans. For instance, he so badly wants to "mend" the early abandonment by his mother that after his discharge from the Marine Corps, he becomes her caretaker. The tattooing of his name on his shoulder symbolizes his idealized feelings for his father. Mr. Evans' attachment traumas contribute to his feelings reflected in his AAP. He tells us that he is unworthy of his parents' care, worthless as a person, and frightened by their unwillingness and inability to protect him.

The deactivation in the Cemetery, Corner, and Ambulance stories evidences Mr. Evans' primary defensive attempt to regulate these feelings. He shows that he relies on authority and social roles, negative evaluation, and avoidance. These representations of self parallel Mr. Evans' behaviors and the need for authority within his own life to create some sense of stability. The intimate and attachment-activating context of bedtime that has been difficult and confusing for Mr. Evans in his own life leads him to shut down describing these interactions in his Bed story. His story describes a structured interaction between the mother and child reading a story and the child falling asleep. Additionally, he relies upon a script-like approach to these interactions to remove any sense of intimacy or mother-child warmth.

In Mr. Evans' own life, he focuses on achievement in the military as a means for containing his feelings of dysregulation. For example, as we noted earlier, he aspired to join an elite faction of the Marines "to make something of himself" and stated that he did well in several training programs even though he did not complete them.

In addition to achievement, the authoritative nature of school and the military are designed to structure, focus, and contain his disorganized world. Similarly, with increased difficulties with life stressors after leaving the military, Mr. Evans becomes reliant upon the court system, VA services, and social workers to provide a structure within his chaotic world.

Other evidence of Mr. Evans' deactivation is manifest in his preference to work by himself as a means for avoiding personal interactions and the potential to let someone down. Finally, Mr. Evans' increased alcohol usage can be viewed as an attempt to anesthetize himself from his pain and the multiplicative horrors of war in concert with his earlier life traumas.

Mr. Evans is in a state of Unresolved chronic mourning. His inability to mourn attachment figure failed protection as a child is compounded by adult traumas during his deployment and Veteran years. This litany of trauma has left him both at risk for mental health and relationship difficulties. Mr. Evans finds himself with deep feelings of guilt, self-reproach, and shame. These feelings likely underlie his current experiences of depression and PTSD. Mr. Evans' AAP suggests a path for the future by building agency, his ability to engage in connected relationships, developing more adaptive emotion regulation strategies, and naming and addressing his Unresolved attachment traumas that carry forward significant risk.

Mr. Evans' responses on the AAP help shed light on possible mechanisms in which Unresolved attachment classification may manifest itself in ways that would dampen clinical improvements in an EBT for Veterans with PTSD. Mr. Evans' dysregulation disrupts his thinking and emotion regulation abilities. This disruption contributes to maladaptive coping strategies while also facilitating depression-related feelings of helplessness and hopelessness. Consistent with his reported difficulties using emotion regulation strategies under duress (via the DERS), Mr. Evans struggled to stay on task, identify his emotional states, or recognize that intense negative feelings are not permanent. Self-awareness of emotional states is a critical skill for patients in EBTs to establish records of negative thoughts that accompany intense negative feelings evoked during treatment. Nevertheless, that insight is fundamentally lacking in Unresolved veterans with PTSD. Rather than experiencing a progressive sense of a corrective learning experience during weekly therapeutic confrontations with traumatic content, Veterans with Unresolved attachments would likely experience an increase in disorganized distress, causing a greater likelihood of drop out from and non-compliance with treatment. Finally, most EBTs for PTSD are not relationship focused but consider symptomatology over broad domains of functioning. As such, neither the distinct impact of attachment trauma from those experienced in combat nor the specific impacts of trauma on relational functioning are pursued.

Treatment

At the VA, Mr. Evans received Cognitive Processing Therapy (CPT) for PTSD. As a manualized evidence-based therapy, each session's agenda is mapped out so that the clinician guides the expectations and therapy topics of 12 weekly sessions. CPT is predicated on cognitive theories related to how negative beliefs inform and drive negative emotions. The early treatment objective is to identify these thoughts in the patient's life experiences and note how they relate to emotional reactions. The therapist then highlights how negative thoughts and feelings fuel avoidance behaviors that strengthen the negative thoughts and feelings through the principle of negative reinforcement. For CPT in particular, negative beliefs or distorted cognitions are referred to as "stuck points." These stuck points usually involve distortions regarding themes of safety, trust, power/control, esteem, and intimacy. For example, "Bad things happen to bad people, so I must have deserved this. Therefore, I feel intense guilt and depression." CPT therapists ask the patient to write out their trauma narrative, describing how they believe the event happened and the thoughts and feelings it elicits. The therapist then engages the patient with their narrative, helping them identify the stuck points in it, and uses Socratic dialogue to challenge these beliefs with more rational alternatives. The patient is asked to revise the narrative over the 12 sessions and read it in between sessions as nightly homework. Ultimately, the therapist challenges the patient to re-engage previously avoided thoughts, feelings, and actions to break the negative reinforcement learning.

Once sober, Mr. Evans was able to identify the guilt and other symptoms he was experiencing with greater levels of intensity than while drinking. He chose as his primary trauma the death of his teammate and could report that his preference for working alone was an avoidance of engaging with new people. From a CPT perspective, the objectives of treatment were to (1) challenge Mr. Evans' distorted belief that he was responsible for his colleague's death ("because I wasn't there with them working with them, I could've seen something – I could've done something"); (2) demonstrate that Mr. Evans was capable of tolerating excruciating negative feelings of mourning and loss, without the use of alcohol; and (3) identify that re-engaging with new relationships and opportunities carry with it an acceptable amount of risk of vulnerability and potential for non-catastrophic loss or rejection.

Unfortunately, Mr. Evans struggled to keep his appointments and engage in the required weekly therapeutic homework assignments. The 12 CPT sessions usually scheduled over eight to twelve weeks were completed over six months. He frequently missed appointments without notice and often took weeks to re-establish contact. Notably, his non-compliance began with the request to write out his trauma narrative during the third session. He noted ongoing custody issues with the mother of his first child and the dissolution of his relationship with the mother of his second child contributing to his difficulties in maintaining treatment. The expectation that he was reviewing his trauma narrative in between sessions was laid aside as the therapist attempted to confront Mr. Evans's distorted beliefs during each session. By the end of the six months, he finished CPT. However, his session-by-session self-report PTSD symptom scores remained unchanged until the final session, which indicated a significant 20-point decrease. While that is a considerable decrease, his score was still at a clinically significant elevation. He passed enough sobriety tests combined with attendance in an ongoing support group that the judge declared Mr. Evans had graduated from the court program. It was recommended that Mr. Evans utilize additional VA treatment to support his sobriety and focus on relapse prevention, to which he initially agreed. However, he failed to answer the multiple follow-up contacts by his PTSD treatment provider. His final court report listed him as continuing to have a PTSD diagnosis.

An alternative attachment treatment approach

It is likely that directly starting treatment with the attachment trauma itself would have been too overwhelming for Mr. Evans, much as writing and reviewing his trauma narrative was in CPT. Characterized by poor emotion regulation skills, Mr. Evans does not have the capacity to "face" his trauma. Mr. Evans' ability to complete CPT, albeit in an incredibly prolonged fashion, was "effective," likely because the slow pace allowed him to metabolize his distress while relying on the authoritative structure placed around him by the court. The judge, court, threats of jail time, and stints in jail were necessary to structure Mr. Evans' sobriety and keep him engaged in treatment. This needed structure was consistent with his defensive deactivation on the AAP. As such, teaching Mr. Evans emotion regulation skills and mindfulness may be necessary steps toward his ultimate therapeutic goals. Ongoing alcohol relapse prevention support would also likely be vital for him as life stressors often lead to relapse.

Notably, while Mr. Evans completed his CPT program, we hypothesize that his Unresolved attachment classification may well account for and contribute to the disrupted nature of treatment and difficulties with treatment compliance. Mr. Evans's traumas are embedded in early parental and interpersonal loss; however, CPT addresses psychopathology by focusing on the level of present-day thoughts and cognitions. Without addressing the underlying attachment traumas that likely undergird Mr. Evans' subsequent difficulties, it is unlikely that any lasting symptom improvement would ensue. From this perspective, the treatment goal becomes addressing the attachment trauma that lies at the core of his difficulties. A helpful approach would be to build a relationship hierarchy that addresses interpersonal issues with current relationships, beginning with the least threatening and difficult ones and progressing up the intensity hierarchy much as one would with a fear hierarchy in Prolonged Exposure. For instance, beginning with his relationships with his legal caseworker and VA therapist might be a good starting point. Given Mr. Evans's inability to engage consistently with treatment in the past, likely in part due to his hesitancy to engage in interpersonal relationships with people, building relationships in a safe setting and helping Mr. Evans to see the value of doing so would be a critical first step. Moving on to provide him with opportunities in the work context to have non-threatening successful relationships would then follow. These supported interventions would help Mr. Evans develop successful and fulfilling relationships. Mr. Evans must identify how core trust, abandonment, and worthiness of care and love are central to his being. Then he would be able to address current romantic relationships, his desire to be a good father, and finally, how his history of attachment relationships often left him feeling unsafe and in pain.

Another port of entry for treatment may be Mr. Evans' stated desire to serve as a good father to his children. Given Mr. Evans's history of attachment trauma and the chronic unresolved nature of his trauma, parenting is likely to be particularly challenging for Mr. Evans. The caregiving system appears to consolidate as the individual transitions to parenthood (George & Solomon, 2008), shifting the focus from Mr. Evans' attachment relationships to his relationships with his children. Attachment-based parent-child interventions that allow Mr. Evans to re-evaluate his attachment experiences, as well as their subsequent influences on his abilities to serve as a caregiver to his children, may be a critical opportunity for addressing his attachment traumas and moving forward. Attachment-based interventions such as the Circle of Security (Powell et al., 2009) and ABC (Dozier et al., 2018) are designed to increase parental sensitivity and child security. However, these interventions can work in both directions, parent to child and parent to their past. As such, intervention with the caregiving system may also potentiate shifts in parent attachment representations or minimally open the door for greater understanding and awareness of Mr. Evans' parents' failures. While this realization may not be sufficient for creating security, it is plausible that they may provide Mr. Evans with a platform to begin to mourn his experiences of failed protection. Mourning would fortify Mr. Evans' defenses and regulate representations of self to help him develop organized approaches not only to his children but also to his life.

Conclusion

The process for young Marines to be selected in Recon is arduous. The warning that pain, misery, and suffering await those who earn the

Recon title sets the appropriate expectation that the process requires a heightened focus, self-sacrifice, and dedication toward the singular goal of achievement. Some of the skills required for this job are enduring suffering while continuing forward, ignoring pains that may otherwise distract or disorient the Marine, and accepting misery for prolonged periods. The reward for such hardship comes in the fellowship and brotherhood experienced with other Recon Marines. The relationships between Recon Marines enable resilience to the traumas of war. In Mr. Evans' case, his dysregulated ability to make sense of emotional states, engage and maintain efforts to his goals, and develop successful relationships are at the opposite spectrum for what these Marines required. A Reconnaissance saying is: "Never above, never below, always beside you." Such an interpersonal stance is meaningful in its potential value of intimacy, absent roles of authority or servitude. The possible resilience gained from such a personal invitation may well guide future therapeutic interventions.

Notes

1 Italics = defenses; bold = trauma.
2 Italics = defenses; bold = trauma; underline = capacity to act
3 Italics = defenses
4 Italics = defenses; bold = trauma

References

Beck, A. T., Steer, R. A., & Brown, G. (1996). *Beck depression inventory–II.* APA PsycTests. https://doi.org/10.1037/t00742-000

Dozier, M., Bernard, K., & Roben, C. K. P. (2018). Attachment and biobehavioral catch-up. In H. Steele & M. Steele (Eds.), *Handbook of attachment-based interventions* (pp. 27–49). Guilford Press.

Foa, E. B., & Kozak, M. J. (1998). Clinical applications of bioinformational theory: Understanding anxiety and its treatment. *Behavior Therapy, 29*(4), 675–690. https://doi.org/10.1016/S0005–7894(98)80025-7.

Garbarino, J., Kostelny, K., & Dubrow, N. (1991). What children can tell us about living in danger. *American Psychologist, 46*(4), 376–383. https://doi.org/10.1037/0003-066X.46.4.376

George, C., & Solomon, J. (2008). The caregiving system: A behavioral systems approach to parenting. In J. Cassidy & P. R. Shaver (Eds.), *Handbook of attachment: Theory, research, and clinical applications* (2nd ed., pp. 833–856). Guilford Press.

Gratz, K. L., & Roemer, L. (2004). Multidimensional assessment of emotion regulation and dysregulation: Development, factor structure, and initial validation of the difficulties in emotion regulation scale. *Journal of Psychopathology and Behavioral Assessment, 26*(1), 41–54. https://doi.org/10.1023/B:JOBA.0000007455.08539.94

Horowitz, L. M., Rosenberg, S. E., Baer, B. A., Ureño, G., & Villaseñor, V. S. (1988). Inventory of interpersonal problems: psychometric properties and clinical applications. *Journal of Consulting and Clinical Psychology, 56*(6), 885. doi.org/10.1037/0022–006X.56.6.885

Litz, B. T., Berke, D. S., Kline, N. K., Grimm, K., Rusowicz-Orazem, L., Resick, P. A., Foa, E. B., Wachen, J. S., McLean, C. P., Dondanville, K. A., Borah, A. M., Roache, J. D., Young-McCaughan, S., Yarvis, J. S., Mintz, J., & Peterson, A. L. (2019). Patterns and predictors of change in trauma-focused treatments for war-related posttraumatic stress disorder. *Journal of Consulting and Clinical Psychology, 87*(11), 1019–1029. https://doi.org/10.1037/ccp0000426

Powell, B., Cooper, G., Hoffman, K., & Marvin, R. S. (2009). The circle of security. In C. H. Zeanah, Jr. (Ed.), *Handbook of infant mental health* (3rd ed., pp. 450–467). Guilford Press.

Steenkamp, M. M., Litz, B. T., & Marmar, C. R. (2020). First-line psychotherapies for military-related PTSD. *Journal of the American Medical Association, 323*(7), 656–657. https://doi.org/10.1001/jama.2019.20825

Weathers, F. W., Litz, B. T., Keane, T. M., Palmieri, P. A., Marx, B. P., & Schnurr, P. P. (2013). The PTSD Checklist for *DSM-5* (PCL-5). Scale available from the National Center for PTSD at www.ptsd.va.gov.

Part 3

Adult psychotherapy and assessment

8 From Unresolved to earned Secure attachment

The AAP as a powerful clinical tool in psychotherapy

Stephen E. Finn

I have previously written about the therapeutic benefits of giving clients feedback about the results of the Adult Attachment Projective Picture System (AAP; George & West, 2012) in the middle of long-term psychotherapy (Finn, 2011). This chapter will explain and illustrate how the AAP picture stimuli are powerful therapeutic tools in and of themselves, and how they provide opportunities for clinicians to help clients reintegrate and reconsolidate implicit emotions and memories tied to their problems in living. I begin by introducing the woman whose story I detail in this chapter; my initial engagement involved a couples' assessment.

Couples' therapeutic assessment and initial AAP administration

I first met "Carole," when she and her husband of 38 years, "Bill," came to Austin for a couples' Therapeutic Assessment (TA). (See Finn, 2015, for a detailed description of couples TA.) At the time, Carole was 65 years old, and Bill was 70. I learned that Bill had precipitously "left" Carole three months earlier while she was away on a trip by emailing that he was deeply unhappy with the marriage and wanted to end it. He had accused Carole of no longer caring about him, treating him like an "appliance," and asked her to stay away until he could move out the house. Carole had been caught off guard completely and was devastated. She had stayed with her adult son for a week before returning home and was unable to function for several weeks. She sought outpatient psychiatric care and gradually got back on her feet but was still confused about why Bill had left and whether there was any hope of reconciliation. Bill had heard about couples' TA from his individual psychotherapist and broached the idea with Carole, telling her that he was willing to postpone a divorce and work on their relationship for one year. After some negotiations by phone and email (during which I asked both of them to sign an agreement that the TA results would not be used in any future legal proceedings), the couple arrived in Austin for several weeks of intensive psychological testing combined with individual and couples' psychotherapy.

DOI: 10.4324/9781003215431-11

Although I will focus on Carole for most of this chapter, first let me summarize the couples TA. At the beginning of the process, I asked Bill and Carole to pose questions they wanted to have addressed through the assessment. Carole was mainly focused on understanding the relationship rupture, asking, *What is it that I failed to provide Bill that led to his needing to leave?* and *Is there something I did that made Bill think I wouldn't be devastated by his leaving?* Bill seemed more focused on building an apologia for himself, asking, *Why did I leave the way that I did?* and *Was there something in the relationship that led to my leaving without a face-to-face discussion?* All these questions seemed very apt to me, as both Bill and Carole described being very much in love at the beginning of their relationship, successfully raising children together, and supporting each other in highly successful careers. Bill complained that in recent years, Carole had become increasingly involved in her work and friends and emotionally distant from him, for example, not giving him a card or gift on Valentine's Day. Carole said she was still in love with Bill, had been unaware of his being unhappy in the marriage, but that he too had become more emotionally committed to other relationships over the previous three to four years. Bill's withdrawal bothered Carole to some extent, and she told of speaking to him about her feelings but dropping the topic when he got defensive. Still, Carole had never considered that the marriage was in danger.

During the TA, both individuals took a series of psychological tests, including the MMPI-2-RF (Ben-Porath & Tellegen, 2008), Rorschach (R-PAS, Meyer et al., 2011), Early Memory Procedure (Bruhn, 1992a, 1992b), and AAP. Bill's and Carole's MMPI-2-RF profiles were very similar, showing little or no emotional distress or disturbance and reflecting their high level of functioning overall. There were indications Carole had difficulty standing up for herself in personal relationships, while Bill could easily "mow people down" to get what he wanted. Interestingly, both of their Rorschach (R-PAS) protocols revealed a great deal of underlying distress and disturbance, which each of them kept out of awareness with exceptional psychological resources and coping mechanisms. Bill appeared to be quite narcissistically vulnerable and could be expected to respond with aggression and distorted thinking when he felt shame. There were suggestions that Bill had a great deal of unresolved trauma. Carole appeared to be highly emotionally sensitive, and likely to defer to others in close relationships. She also appeared to be managing a number of underlying painful emotions, which was not unexpected given the marital crisis.

The pattern of results fit with information that began to emerge from our interviews with the couple. Bill reiterated his narrative that Carole had "given him the cold shoulder" over the previous four to five years of the marriage, devoting herself to work and friends and avoiding physical affection and sex. Thus, he had sought friendship and comfort elsewhere. Bill admitted he had not spoken to Carole about his unhappiness but could not explain why, and he had no idea why Carole might have pulled back from their relationship. At first, Carole denied that she had been more distant from Bill, pointing to functional ways she still did a lot for him and their relationship. However, gradually, she began to see that she may have "put up a wall" without realizing it. For example, Carole no longer talked to Bill about her work because he got angry if she did not follow his advice, and she stopped sharing her successes because typically he would grow jealous and pout. Also, Carole avoided certain social situations as a couple, because if she expressed opinions different from his, Bill would become enraged, demeaning, and berate her in the car on the way home. Last, Carole admitted she avoided sex and other physical contact with Bill, as he was often rough and ignored her pleas that she was in pain. Bill confirmed Carole's account of these things in our conjoint sessions but seemed to have "forgotten" most of the incidents where he had acted badly until he was reminded. Even then, Bill had difficulty appreciating the effect of his behavior on Carole, often "turning the tables" to complain about her. I also found it very challenging in our individual sessions to help Bill explore what might underlie his aggressive and controlling outbursts; he kept explaining that this type of behavior had made him successful in his business, that he valued it, and he had difficulty going any deeper.

At this point in the TA, the three of us were faced with several major puzzles:

(1) Why had Bill not spoken up directly about his desire for more attention and affection from Carole? What provoked his demeaning and aggressive behavior?
(2) Why had Carole not stood up to Bill about his aggressive and demeaning behavior? Why had she stayed, and how had she kept herself from feeling unhappy with the marriage?

I was aware that cultural norms and gender-role expectations were relevant, especially in Bill's and Carole's generation. Carole had been "taught" that women should accept bad treatment from men and not confront them, although clearly she had defied this model in her work life. Bill had been "taught" that vulnerability and emotional longing were shameful for men, and that women were supposed to support men materially and emotionally and provide sex whenever it was requested. Although these cultural factors were compelling, I felt that more was at stake. And so, I asked Bill and Carole to complete the Early Memory Procedure and AAP.

AAP results

Bill's AAP stories were lengthy and full of confusion and uncertainty and trauma markers. The resulting classification was Unresolved, and his main regulating defense was cognitive disconnection, with several unresolved segregated systems in his response to the Cemetery scene. This story involved a man who felt isolated and guilty following a loss for which he was partly responsible. None of Bill's stories depicted attachment figures who were helpful, comforting, or loving, and instead parents were depicted as potential sources of fear and danger. Although I was aware that the unresolved story to Cemetery might reflect Bill's guilt over leaving Carole, I suspected there was early attachment trauma also (see Chapter 4). The picture of his childhood that emerged from his early memories was of alcoholic and neglectful parents involved in an ongoing marital "war"; Bill's emotional needs had not been attended to and frequently he had assumed adult responsibilities in the family. As a teen, Bill had felt alienated and inadequate relative to his peers, but later achieved social success by "learning to fight" and becoming a "bull" who could not be stopped. Although Bill could be charming and engaging when he was regulated, he was vulnerable to shame and to getting disorganized, at which point he could be quite aggressive. I suspected that for much of their relationship, Carole had supported Bill's self-esteem and kept him organized; similarly, he had provided a stable base for her. However, as Carole became more successful and independent, Bill felt abandoned emotionally, but was too ashamed to directly and vulnerably ask for attention. Instead, he had alternated between withdrawal and attacking.

Carole's AAP had many classic dismissing themes, with characters who coped with difficult feelings by achieving and "carrying on." This was her story to Window:[1]

This is me... this is a girl...alone looking out the window. Looking for something *she doesn't know* what she is	Disconnect
looking for. She's sad. And she's alone. And *doesn't know*	Disconnect
what to do. Before she got to the window, she *I don't know*, was talking to someone in her family and was told to go away, go play or something like that. After she looks out the window for a while she leaves and <u>goes to her room</u>	Agency: action
<u>and picks up a book</u>. ... Why did the picture make me	Deactivate
sad? (laugh) mean it did (sign) She's thinking I have to take care of myself and *How do I do that? I just don't know...*	Disconnect
there's nobody there who's gonna take care of me. I have to take care of myself, whatever that means. And I don't mean in a physical needs way, but *I don't know* emotional	Disconnect
way I think.	

Three of Carole's stories contained evidence of attachment trauma, and the overall classification of Carole's AAP was Unresolved with deactivation as the main regulating defense. The Unresolved classification was because of her story to the Departure scene. The story clearly reflected her experience of Bill's ending their marriage three months earlier.[2]

This is a story of a husband who's leaving his wife. He's got his *suit* on. And she's got her head slightly bowed and he's telling her something maybe why he's leaving. And she is looking sad	Deactivate
and **bereft**. And he looks like of *galvanized*. Ready to leave.	Trauma
She turns around and has a kind of **stunned** look on her face.	Trauma
She's got this big house and these kids and now she has to take care of it. All of it. And she's thinking *What happened. I don't understand. What?* And he says, "You know I'm leaving	Disconnect
because I can't live with you anymore. You're not what I need, and I just want to get away." That sounds familiar doesn't it? Before he got up and got dressed and as he usually does and	
she kind of *snoozed* a little bit to give him space to get dressed.	Deactivate
He then pulled out the suitcase and is *throwing the suitcase*.	Disconnect
And she's going, *Are you going on a business trip you didn't tell me about?* He said, "No, I'm not. I'm leaving you." And	
she is in **complete and utter shock. What?** He carried the[3]	Trauma
suitcases downstairs and was all feeling good about himself	
and *oblivious to what she was thinking or feeling* 'cause he	Disconnect
really didn't care. He got in his car and said, "You should go in the house. The kids are about to get up," and he drove off.	

As is evident, the segregated system in this story was not resolved. The woman is dysregulated (shock) and nobody comes to her aid. The man leaves her in this psychological state.

Carole's story to the subsequent picture, Bench, was also full of trauma. It concerned a woman who had received "some bad news" and was "in despair...alone...helpless." She was sitting down because "if she got up, she would probably fall down on the floor." In this story, however, the segregated systems were contained by Capacity to Act; the woman "pulled herself together" and went about her daily activities, even though she was full of despair and loss. I surmised that although Carole was functioning better than she had right after receiving Bill's email, her attachment system was still vulnerable to disorganization. From my discussions with Bill and Carole, I hypothesized that Carole's attachment status prior to the recent crisis was probably Dismissing, at least in recent years. Bill's description of Carole's "giving him the cold shoulder" fit exactly with what spouses of Dismissing partners experience (Tatkin, 2009). Also, Carole's not being in touch with her own dissatisfaction with the marriage and equating the functional care she did in the relationship with "showing love" fit with her having adopted a dismissing adaption.

Importantly, I suspected that Carole's dismissing defenses and vulnerability to disorganization predated her experiences with Bill. I knew that she had been married and divorced previously, and that her first husband had been emotionally abusive and denigrating. Eventually Carole had left him, finished her graduate studies, and married Bill. Also, although Carole had initially described her childhood as benign and her parents as "typical for their era," in her early memories and from our discussions

I learned that her father had been a highly narcissistic, distant, and demeaning man. Her mother, although caring and highly intelligent, had submerged herself in the marriage, putting much of her energy into tending to the household, supporting her husband's career, and both modeling and teaching Carole never to oppose her father. Carole described her mother as having "shut down" in the face of her father's derision and dominance. We agreed that this had left her mother less emotionally available to her, and this fit with Carole's story to the Bed scene of the AAP. In Carole's account, a mother is lecturing her son at bedtime about some "transgression" he committed during the day. The boy is distressed and crying and reaching to the mother for comfort, calling "mommy, mommy." The mother "withholds her affection" until she is finished speaking and then gives the child "a brief hug" and tells him to lay down and go to sleep.

As Carole and I discussed her AAP stories and early memories, she began to revise her understanding of her childhood and to solve the previously mentioned puzzles about the marriage, that is, how she had been able to put her own unhappiness with Bill aside and "carry on," and why she had not taken a stronger stance with Bill about his abusive behavior. Carole came to see that she had followed in her mother's footsteps in many ways, except that Carole had been able to build a life outside of her marriage, which in the end indirectly led to Bill's leaving. As the couples' TA moved toward its end, Carole had clearly grown a great deal in her self-understanding and seemed committed to repairing her marriage with Bill.

Conclusion of the couples' therapeutic assessment

However, Bill was in a different place. As mentioned earlier, I felt he had a hard time facing the personal issues that had emerged during the assessment: his neglectful and traumatized childhood, his vulnerability to shame, and his tendency to intimidate and control others to keep himself regulated. In an individual session with me, Bill confessed that he had never intended to use the couples' TA to come back together with Carole. Rather, his goal was to help Carole "understand his position" better so as to have a "less contentious divorce." I saw this disclosure as a test of whether I would side with him against Carole and told Bill I would not keep his intentions private from Carole. So, in our next conjoint session, Bill told Carole had no intention of reconciling and that he had invited her to Austin on false premises. Carole, understandably, was furious about being misled. Also, she managed to get Bill to admit that he was already sexually involved with another woman, which led to her also wishing to end the marriage. As the TA closed, I hoped that it had served as a kind of "postmortem" on the relationship, and that Bill and Carole better understood what had gone wrong in their marriage.

I suggested that each of them seek support as they finalized their divorce, and I agreed to help Carole find an individual therapist in her area to continue the work she had begun during the TA.

My work with Carole after the couples' therapeutic assessment

I used various professional contacts to identify potential therapists for Carole after she returned home, even interviewing some of them myself. Carole ended up having two to three sessions with two different therapists, both of whom she did not find very helpful. Then, she contacted me and asked if I would work with her, proposing we have regular virtual sessions interspersed with her coming to Austin several times a year for intensive work. I asked that Carole allow me to check with Bill, and he verified that he no longer wanted my services for either individual or couples' sessions, and said he hoped I could help Carole. So, approximately three months following the conclusion of the couples' TA, Carole and I began weekly virtual psychotherapy sessions.

Early phase of psychotherapy

Initially, our work centered on supporting Carole through the separation and divorce negotiations with Bill and making sense of all the intense feelings that were coming up. Although Carole understood intellectually that Bill and she could not stay together, she kept experiencing a great deal of grief about the relationship and longing to be with him. When this happened, she would become quite self-critical about her age and appearance and then fall into despair, envisioning herself being alone for the rest of her life. I sat with Carole in her grief without trying to cheer her up, validated that the end of the marriage was a huge loss, and tried to help her understand that her painful feelings were partly about Bill, but also probably about other attachment relationships. At my encouragement, Carole brought into therapy sessions a number of photos of herself and her family from when she was a child. We noticed how depressed her mother looked in all the photos, and how Carole herself looked shut down and tense after about age 5. I led her in some enactments in which we talked to "little Carole," a technique I had adapted from the Ideal Parent Figure Method (Brown & Elliot, 2016; Parra et al., 2017). These dialogues helped Carole become more aware of her deactivating attachment strategies. At first, when asked to offer reassurance and comfort, Carole would simply urge her younger self to "hang in there" and "be strong." With my help, she began to name and reflect the inner pain we saw, and to say "I know you are hurting. I love you and will not leave you; I will always be there for you." Also, Carole was able to use some of these phrases with herself at night, when her longing and despair became overwhelming, and this helped calm her to some extent. I felt there was more we could do if we met in person, and Carole and I agreed she would come to Austin for some intensive work. Her main question for our sessions was: "Why am I still struggling with all this grief when I know I don't want to be with Bill? And what can I do about this excruciating longing?" I hoped to help Carole understand the extent of her early attachment trauma so that she could have more compassion for her struggles at the time.

Return to Austin and second AAP administration

Thirteen months after the initial couples' assessment, Carole came to Austin for three days. We met for six three-hour sessions, during which I repeated the MMPI-2-RF, Rorschach, and AAP, and we discussed them. As mentioned earlier, Carole's original MMPI-2-RF had shown very little emotional distress, so it was interesting that on retest somewhat more pain was visible. The MMPI-2-RF also suggested that Carole was now more in touch with self-protective anger, which fit with my observations of how assertively she was handling the divorce negotiations with Bill. The R-PAS profile was much improved also, showing even stronger coping resources than on the original testing and more capacity for connecting to others.

However, the main event of our sessions that weekend centered on the AAP. The coded protocol showed substantial changes in Carole's attachment representations. This time there were no unresolved segregated systems in any of the stories, the number of trauma indicators had decreased. Instead of the original Unresolved classification, the current AAP classification was Dismissing, Failed Mourning (see Chapter 4). Also, she demonstrated relationship Synchrony integration in response to the dyadic pictures (see Chapter 1). In Carole's first Bed story, the mother withheld affection and lectured her son about a transgression. In her new Bed story, "...[he] extends his arms to her saying 'I love you, mommy, I love you' and she grabs him and holds him and says 'I love you. I love you too.' And then she kind of tickles him a little bit and they lie down and laugh together and snuggle for a little while..." I suspected this shift in Carole's representation of attachment was a direct result of the psychotherapy sessions in which we had helped Carole "talk" to her distressed younger self in a soothing way.

Although these changes were all positive, I was very struck by Carole's story to Window[4]:

This little girl was walking through the living room and stopped to look out the window and she sees the big, beautiful tree. And she *wonders* about *its mystery and*	Disconnect
what it was like when it was a tiny little tree and how	Dereal – surreal
it grew to be so big and how old it was and	

everything it had seen and how long it would be there.
And she's kind of marveling at the tree. And she feels
good about that. It's kind of like *between her and*
the tree. She thinks about just kind of *being one with*
the tree. And then once she is finished thinking about
the tree she turned and <u>went into the kitchen to have</u>   Agency: action
<u>breakfast</u>. She feels good about the tree. It's ancient but
at the same time not. It makes her feel good about it and
somehow it makes her feel good about herself too. She
makes plans <u>to go sit under the tree</u>.   Agency: action

I remembered that Carole's previous story to this picture was of a little girl who was sad and alone and didn't know what to do with herself and so used deactivation ("picking up a book") to regulate her attachment system. I surmised that this time, the picture had activated the same kind of attachment distress in Carole, but she had not managed to deactivate, and so instead had ended regulating in derealization (i.e., depersonalization). I knew derealization was a dissociative coping mechanism associated with severe attachment trauma. In our next session, I decided to discuss my thoughts with Carole.

I showed the Window picture and read Carole her story. We appreciated together how the girl in the story had "made herself" feel good via her imagination. I asked Carole what the girl would have felt if she hadn't been able to fantasize.

CAROLE: I think she's feeling very alone and maybe abandoned but focusing on the tree helps her feel good.

STEVE: Yes, how creative! Do you think that same strategy ever worked for you?

CAROLE: I think it did when I was young. Then later I learned how to achieve in order to feel better.

STEVE: That seems right. I wonder, are you willing to do an experiment with me now?

CAROLE: Yes.

STEVE: Can you look hard at the picture, then close your eyes and imagine you are that little girl and there is no tree there to think about or activity you can do? Describe what you are feeling...

CAROLE: *(Long pause)* It's awful! I see black all around me. I am so scared that I want to scream, but I can't make a noise.

I asked Carole to "stay there" a bit longer. She nodded yes and fell silent. Her face looked anguished and frightened. Then Carole suddenly opened her eyes. I saw terror in her eyes and asked her to talk about what she had experienced. She described the feeling of being in a "black hole," completely alone and terrified, with nothing or no one to "grab onto." I asked if she would be willing to go back into that place one more time, but with me physically holding her hand. She gulped and nodded yes. I moved my chair closer and took her hand, she closed her eyes, and began to sob.

CAROLE: This is awful. I feel as if I'm floating in space. I am so incredibly scared. *(Crying hard.)* I don't think I can stand this.
STEVE: Squeeze my hand! I'm right here. You're in this awful place but I've got you. Stay with the feelings but listen to my words. Do you hear me?
CAROLE: Yes *(very softly)*.
STEVE: I know you are terrified. I know you feel alone. But I'm here. You're going to get through this. You've touched into something that is deep inside, an old feeling, an experience from long ago that was more than you could handle on your own. But you're not alone anymore. I'm here. You're going to come out of this, and you're grown up now. This feeling is old. You survived it. Now you can always reach out to others. You can take care of this scared part of you and others will help.

Carole gradually grew calmer, opened her eyes, and looked confused. But almost immediately she grew curious about what had just happened, saying, "I never knew that was in there! What happened?" I told her I wanted her to come back fully to the room and then we would talk about her experience. She went to the restroom and washed her face, returned, and we talked for another 30 minutes. I explained that I thought she had re-experienced an old attachment trauma, where she was alone and terrified and overwhelmed. She was in awe of the experience and what it meant. She agreed it was very likely that her mother had been so depressed at times that she had been left absolutely alone as a small child. After a while, I noticed Carole's eyes drooping, and when I asked, she admitted she was exhausted. We agreed to stop, she left and went to her hotel knowing she could call me that night if she needed to. When we met the next morning, Carole said she had eaten something light, then fallen into bed and slept deeply all night. She said she had awoken feeling calm and "freer," as if she had cast off a burden she hadn't even known she was carrying.

We spent the rest of the closing session discussing the meaning of the experience with the Window story the day before. I again explained that I believed Carole had suffered severe attachment trauma as a child, and that this was why she was still struggling with painful feelings now that Bill was gone. I interpreted that these feelings were why she had been unable to leave Bill, or even let herself know she was unhappy in the marriage, because there was no way she could have faced them on her own. Carole understood this and seemed more forgiving of herself for staying with Bill and for longing for him after the relationship ended, saying, "I now see it wasn't Bill I was longing for, but for someone to care for me."

Carole was also more accepting of why she was not "all better" at that point in time. I promised her that we would continue to work on these issues in psychotherapy, and that I had ideas of what might help her more.

Next year of psychotherapy and third AAP administration

Carole and I continued to meet virtually for psychotherapy after she returned home, and we both noticed a shift that we attributed to our work in Austin with the AAP stimulus. She continued to feel freer and had more energy. She began to explore dating, and we spent sessions talking about those experiences, and in particular about one man she felt very attracted to who would pursue her and then disappear, only to contact her again and seek closeness. Over time, Carole became more and more skeptical of this man, and could see that he was not available as a partner because of his obvious ambivalence about intimacy. Carole also began to explore other interests and decided to take graduate courses in religion, a topic she had long wanted to study. I suggested Carole supplement our therapy sessions with some therapeutic body work, as my clinical experience had taught me this was an effective adjunct to therapy in clients with early trauma. Carole had several sessions with a practitioner certified in Somatic Experiencing (Levine, 1997), and these seemed to have a good impact.

A little over three years after the original couples' TA, Carole came to Austin again for three days of in-person sessions, with the goal of our continuing to think about her next growth steps. Once again, we repeated the AAP. To my satisfaction, this time the protocol was classified Secure. I felt this result reflected the good work we had done in therapy and the healing I had seen in Carole over the previous year. This time, there were even more signs of good Synchrony and Connection. Her security was evident in Corner[5]:

This little boy is in a corner and being *punished for some infraction*. But he's been holding up his hands, *arguing* with his mother that he shouldn't be in the corner... saying *I didn't do it. I didn't do it*. And he's turning his head, which means probably he may have done it, and he's trying to convince her that he didn't do it. Before she put him in the corner and he's *mad* about it. Claimed he didn't do it. Since he can't convince her, he stays in there the full 10 minutes and his *anger* kind of dissipates because he knows he did it. About the end of the 10 minutes, he calms down and she comes in the room and says, "It's okay, time out is over. And he says, *"I'm sorry." And she says, "Okay, come here."* and he went to her, and *she hugged him and said she loved him* and that sometimes people do bad things but it doesn't mean they're bad and *she loves him. He says, "I love you too, mommy."*	Deactivate
	
	Disconnect
	Deactivate &
	  Agency: action
	
	Disconnect
	
	Disconnect
	
	Agency: haven of
	  safety, repair
	
	Agency: haven of
	  safety, repair

As you can see, there still were a number of attachment defenses present in the story, but these all were in the service of repair and integration. How was this kind of change in Carole's attachment representation reflected in her life? She was more connected to friends, more content with the idea that she might not be partnered again, and more adept at figuring out what she wanted from life and pursuing it. She had decided to seek a graduate degree in religion and was getting top grades in her program. Although Carole could be self-critical of her appearance still, she was doing less of that. And to my eye, she was more alive, more expressive emotionally, and handling a myriad of life challenges with resilience and good judgment. For example, Carole still had some dealings with Bill over joint financial holdings, but she felt little turmoil when he tried to charm or bully her, easily setting limits in a calm but firm manner. In fact, she told me she now felt grateful that Bill had left her, as it had spurred her work with me, and she now was happier in her life than she ever remembered.

Afterthoughts and a brief poem from Carole

Carole and I continue to meet from time to time for virtual therapy sessions. The COVID pandemic has prevented us from seeing each other in person recently, but it has also seemed less urgent to do so. When I talked to Carole about writing this chapter, she was open to my doing so and was very curious. This spurred our discussing important events in the therapy, and in particular Carole's "trip to the black hole" several years back via the AAP Window picture. She said she thought this was a crucial experience in our work together and that coming through that experience had truly shifted much of the grief she had been harboring. I shared with Carole a poem I had come across on therapy by Nayyirah Waheed in her 2013 book *Salt*. It opens with the phrase, "The hard season will split you through..." and describes the anguish and grief that will come up for clients in deep psychotherapy until "the soft season" comes, "to drink all the damage into love" (p. 9). Carole was touched by the poem and thought it beautifully captured her experiences in therapy. She then sent me a new ending, dedicated to me in gratitude of what "we had accomplished together":

> Do not worry,
> you will
> begin to breathe again
> and see
> the colors of joy as
> the pain recedes and is absorbed
> as a wave on the shore.
> Do not worry,

because darkness will become light and
you will forgive yourself as shame washes away.
Do not worry, it will come,
you will recognize the Beloved you are.

Of course, I was moved and grateful, and also felt humbled by the privilege of working with someone like Carole. In addition, I was very thankful for the power of the AAP and eager to tell other clinicians about its power as a tool in psychotherapy.

Notes

1 Italics = defenses; underline = capacity to act
2 Italics = defenses; bold = trauma;
3 Italics = defenses; bold = trauma
4 Italics = defenses; bold = trauma; underline = capacity to act
5 Italics = defenses; underline = capacity to act

References

Brown, D. P., & Elliott, D. S. (2016). *Attachment disturbances in adults: Treatment for comprehensive repair*. Norton.

Bruhn, A. R. (1992a). The early memories procedure: A projective test of autobiographical memory (Part I). *Journal of Personality Assessment, 58*(1), 1–15. https://doi.org/10.1207/s15327752jpa5801_1

Bruhn, A. R. (1992b). The early memories procedure: A projective test of autobiographical memory (Part II). *Journal of Personality Assessment, 58*(2), 326–346. https://doi.org/10.1207/s15327752jpa5802_11

Finn, S. E. (2011). Use of the adult attachment projective picture system (AAP) in the middle of a long-term psychotherapy. *Journal of Personality Assessment, 93*(5), 427–433. https://doi.org/10.1080/00223891.2011.595744

Finn, S. E. (2015). Therapeutic Assessment with couples. *Pratiques Psychologues, 21*(4), 345–373. https://doi.org/10.1016/j.prps.2015.09.008

George, C., & West, M. (2012). *The adult attachment projective picture system: Attachment theory and assessment in adults*. Guilford Press.

Levine, P. (1997). *Waking the tiger: Healing trauma*. North Atlantic Books.

Meyer, G. J., Viglione, D. J., Mihura, J. L., Erard, R. E. & Erdberg, P. (2011). *Rorschach performance assessment system: Administration, coding, interpretation, and technical manual*. Rorschach Performance Assessment System.

Parra, F., George, C., Kalalou, K., & Januel, D. (2017). Ideal parent figure method in the treatment of complex posttraumatic stress disorder related to childhood trauma: A pilot study. *European Journal of Psychotraumatology, 8*(1). https://doi.org/10.1080/20008198.2017.1400879

Tatkin, S. (2009). Addiction to "alone time": Avoidant attachment, narcissism, and a one-person psychology in a two-person psychological system. *The Therapist, 57*, January–February.

Waheed, N. (2013). *Salt*. Published by the author. ISBN-13: 978–1492238287.

9 Embodying attachment
Language and somatic revelations

Talia B. Shafir

This chapter illustrates the Adult Attachment Projective Picture System (AAP), a narrative assessment of attachment as it applies to observations of movement in somatic movement therapy. Movement is at the core of attachment from the very beginning of life. Attachment patterns beginning in infancy are observations of movement (i.e., behavior) and responses to their primary caregivers (e.g., Ainsworth et al., 1978). By age 4, and in adolescence and adulthood, attachment patterns can be derived from "observations" of mental representations, that is, individuals' verbal narratives of attachment story themes or their life stories. Language carries the gestalt of that experience; however, early sensory experiences do not disappear. Non-verbal elements of early experience such as a caregiver's touch, vocal quality, and even breathing patterns contribute to those representations. This chapter shows how pairing body movements with the AAP attachment narrative unearths an embodied perspective for adult therapeutic intervention.

Observation during the administration of the AAP reveals somatic responses to the pictures. The perspective taken here is that we can observe how behaviors that originated in the early years morphed into the movement patterns we see as our clients tell the AAP stories. The body reveals its parallel non-verbal narrative in various kinesthetic cues such as posture and gesture, rhythms, and sensory orientation. Thus, language and body in concert form a powerful partnership to inform this embodied approach. The case study presented in this chapter provides examples of how observation of this partnership contributes to therapeutic change.

The meaning of movement patterns and the AAP narrative

Movement is a form of communication. The first lines of communication in the attachment-caregiving dyad are sensory. Touch and movement are paramount. When distressed, the child's movements (i.e., attachment behaviors) are designed to bring the attachment figure close and communicate their protection needs. The child orients, reaches out, or moves

DOI: 10.4324/9781003215431-12

toward their attachment figure, signaling a need to be picked up, held, comforted, or soothed through contact.

Secure attachment ensues if the child's attachment behavior results in timely and consistent sensitive caregiving responses. The child's movements communicate enjoyment and trust. If not, patterns of tension in the body that accompany caregiving inadequacies are folded into mental representations of insecure attachment. Bodily expressions of need or enjoyment are suppressed and replaced by other movement patterns that parallel defensive process strategies formed from a history of attachment system disruption or traumatic failed protection. Over time, these suppressed developmental movement patterns remain enfolded in the growing complexity of the maturing adult (Tsachor & Shafir, 2017). From a somatic point of view, these movements are as much a part of an individual's attachment pattern as the language of the representational narrative.

Movements are mastered developmentally as we embody our history. A current event, set in a specific context, sensory and dynamically similar to one in the past, elicits patterns shaped at that earlier time (Frank & Labarre, 2011). Identifying and repatterning the accompanying movements and the stage of development from which they physically emanate helps provide a sense of agency and feelings of safety in the face of what had previously been a trigger for distress. Attunement to the physical leads to a portal into the workings of the mind. By giving attention to movement patterns expressed in conjunction with a particular perception of an AAP image, subsequent repatterning can reframe the mental representation presented in the narrative. The AAP provides the implicit context via imagery to address both the mental representation and the physical manifestations of adult attachment status (Shafir, 2019). Working with the body's response can change the mind's perception and encourage learning new movement options. The embodied experience, in turn, can affect change in the status of the attachment system.

The AAP stimulates the attachment system by evoking an experience of the moment instead of describing an event reconstructed from memory. It produces a real-time status report following the client's internal and external input processing that is invaluable from a somatic point of view. The result is a dynamic, developmentally organized lens to address the embodied traces of attachment disruption and developmental trauma.

My interest was to examine the intersection of language and body. To do this, I recorded a video of the AAP administration process capturing as much of the body as possible. Using an app such as Otter.ai that displays the time markers as part of the transcript makes it possible to pinpoint the time signature of the AAP content and defensive processing dimensions (see Chapter 1) as they appear in the narrative. (This is particularly helpful when restricted to a remote video recording.) One can then compare the time markers that match the AAP coding in the written transcript with the timestamps of the movement observation in the video recording. This cross-analysis makes it possible to pinpoint the linguistic trigger of the mental representation together with the somatic pattern(s) that supports it. Figure 9.1 provides a sample of the synchronous pattern of defensive language and body response.

Of therapeutic interest are the body's reactions that deviate from baseline. The baseline is determined by watching the movements during the participant's encounter with the first AAP picture, a neutral image that does not activate the attachment system. With subsequent pictures, the observer notes movement patterns that differ from the participant's average repertoire and the time they occur. This additional information provides an opportunity to incorporate developmental movement resourcing and repatterning into the treatment plan. The somatic contribution to the AAP offers a non-verbal path to the elusive, unprocessed emotional material lodged in the unconscious, the integration of which during treatment is key to achieving therapeutic change.

As seen in Figure 9.1, not every AAP code directly matches a time-stamp of a significant movement. Some notable movements appear before and after codes, possibly signaling an attempt to self-regulate. At other times, an arousal response may initiate at first sight of the picture before the participant starts speaking. Delayed movement can also be a carryover result of the effects triggered by the previous picture, especially if that response included segregated systems (i.e., emotional dysregulation and trauma).

	AAP	Movement Observations
5:49	Receives picture	**5:50** bulges with torso (adds bridge to connect); allows small amount of free flow (breathing deepens)
		5:59 - 6:20 flow fluctuation in chest (intermittent breathing disruptions)
6:24	Disconnection	
6:28	Disconnection	**6:28** repetitive head movement
		6:35 head gesture, down and forward

Figure 9.1 Example of timing comparisons between the AAP attachment defense coding and movement observation notes (Shafir, 2019).

Putting embodiment to use

The chapter case study presents an example of using movement to connect mind and body to affect perceptual, functional change and help initiate a path of emotional resiliency and resources for self-efficacy. As with so many others, this client came to therapy to understand what made her feel hopeless and helpless, value others' needs above her own, and her addictions to substances and abusive relationships. The AAP helped address the origins of these concerns by identifying specific attachment defenses as mental representations that mapped the route to her attachment classification. During storytelling, the body's reactions added information that cut through conscious resistance and illuminated non-verbal elements of attachment defense. Movement patterns evoked by the AAP images offered a glimpse into the sensory origins of explicit and implicit memory (i.e., memory encoded before language developed).

Terri's story: A case study of attachment and movement analysis

Terri, a 57-year-old woman of African American and Native American descent, was born on a military base in Europe, the youngest of three. Her father traveled back and forth on active duty in Vietnam and dealt with his severe PTSD via alcohol and domestic violence. She had a history of childhood physical and emotional abuse perpetrated by both parents. At 5, she spent several weeks in the hospital with a life-threatening injury from a brick thrown at her head by a playmate. At 13, she lost consciousness when her father threw her against a wall in a fit of rage. She witnessed her siblings suffer frequent physical and emotional abuse throughout her childhood.

Terri presented clinically with ongoing cocaine, marijuana, and alcohol addiction. She received a diagnosis of bipolar disorder and ADHD four years before her first visit. Under the continuing supervision of a psychopharmacologist, Terri's treatment included a regimen of varying drug combinations, including lithium, Lamictal, Abilify, Cymbalta, Ritalin, and Ambien.

Terri participated in three and a half years of somatic therapy and two eight to twelve week sessions of residential rehab. I administered the AAP twice during her treatment. Her first classification was Dismissing, Failed Mourning. This classification shows that Terri had significant unmourned attachment trauma and created a deactivating shield, including not grieving the loss of her father who had died 15 months earlier, whom she remembered as abusive and mean. Her body showed muscular tension of the torso, holding of her breath, and spinal rigidity. This shield protected her from unprocessed grief and traumatic pain and anguish (See Chapter 4 for a complete description of Failed Mourning).

Terri's alone stories show the intensity of her feelings of traumatic isolation. Except for Window, the alone stories describe a frightened, devastated, and terrorized self. The only parent figures in these stories are abusive authoritarians. Terri's attempts to disconnect from her experience confuse her ability to specify the identities of the people or events at the source of her melancholy and trauma. Even in Corner, she describes the child's abuse in detail but fails to specify precisely what the child did wrong that elicited abuse. Terri's stories show how she faces her trauma alone, and in two stories (Bench, Corner), regulates by readjusting her body (protective agency). Although she names felt affect, deactivating defenses distance their realization. For example, the character in Bench distances herself from displaying her emotions in public. The man in Cemetery emotionally distances himself from his sadness by intellectualizing his visit to his loved one's grave. The child in Corner succumbs to his punishment and corrects the wrong with compliance, by doing "what he is supposed to do."

Terri's dyadic stories describe relationship insensitivity and failure. The adults in Departure separate in anger. In Bed, Terri's immediate response is to infer that a child is signaling his attachment need to his mother, "hands outstretched, looking as if he wants a hug." She cannot describe maternal sensitivity (the mother's immediate response to the signal). Instead, Terri deactivates the child's need for physical closeness and reinterprets the closeness she desires from her attachment figure to a functional connection (happy that the mother reads a story).

Ambulance is a devastating story of a child and a nurse watching a horrifying life-threatening scene. The narrative reads like a PTSD flashback. Encapsulated in the deactivating armor of social role management (a comforting nurse, medical intervention), Terri describes the victim's surreal collapse and flight from reality (derealization) and a child and surrogate caregiver in helpless frozen, suspended animation. "All they can do is sit there and watch... everything buzz around him and listen to the sound of the machines. Just sit there and look at him." This pattern of defense and trauma symbolizes Terri's struggle to self-regulate when no attachment figure is available to offer protection or consolation. Her representational struggle in Ambulance evidences her mistrust and flight from personal relationships.

Embodied punctuation of Teri's AAP narrative: The power of the reach

The visual information captured on video, paired with the AAP codes, identified somatic reactions highlighting the underpinnings of dysfunctional basic developmental movement patterns. Evidence of responses of the autonomic nervous system to unprocessed trauma, that is, intermittent holding of breath, was also visible. When taken as a whole of seven pictures, the AAP movement observations illuminate repetitive bodily reactions, painting a comprehensive picture of the somatic patterning commensurate with activated defense and regulating processes unique to the storyteller. The AAP, then, provides a container not only for revealing the language of mental representation but also for a coherent movement vocabulary.

BodyMind Centering®, a developmentally based somatic healing, well-being, and experiential research system, describes our foundational movement patterns as a sequence of yield, push, reach, grasp, pull, and release (Cohen, 2018). This sequence is one of the strategic lenses through which to observe significant movement patterns that arise during the administration of the AAP. It is not possible in the space allowed here to provide the reader with a complete description of the full spectrum of Terri's somatic responses. The discussion below chronicles accompanying movements of reaching and breathing relevant to several attachment defense processes revealed by her AAP. The discussion then describes somatic intervention demonstrating the power of repatterning a movement phrase that includes a dysfunctional impulse to reach (Shafir, 2015).

Terri was trained to suppress her impulse to reach very early on, under threat of physical punishment. Consistent arm immobility, constricted breathing patterns, and rigid holding of the torso were present throughout the AAP. Combined tension flow patterns formed an attachment defense process by suppressing the reach to avoid punishment and deactivate or shift her conscious attention away from her trauma.

The girl in Window is being punished. Terri's breathing is shallow, and she holds her torso still and upright, reminiscent of a military pose of attention. She reaches out to the therapist as she describes what the girl describes where she would like to be and holds her breath as she faces the reality that her confinement is punishment.[1]

Window	Defense	Movement
A girl standing in her room, looking outside at a scene outside. She looks lonely standing there. She *looks at something that's going on or staring at a tree*. She's thinking, *I wish I could go outside*. But I'm standing here in the house. I have to stay here but *I wish I could be outside*. It's so pretty out there. She has to do something before she goes outside. She may have been *punished*. She's in a room, *wistful, dreaming* about being outside and playing.	Disconnect Disconnect Disconnect Deactivate Disconnect	Shallow breathing; stays in vertical plane; quick, direct hand gestures back and forth. Torso expands to bridge connection with therapist (reaching out) Body stays in vertical plane with minimum movement (military style) Flow fluctuation in chest (intermittent holding of breath)

Terri's upper body restriction and erratic breathing flow into Departure, the next story in the AAP sequence. Her visceral response mirrors the couple's distress, anger, and tension.

Next in Bench, Terri's attachment system is increasingly activated (Buchheim et al., 2006), and we see trauma surfacing in the story theme for the first time.[2]

Bench	Defense	Movement
A *girl or young lady* sits with a **wall** behind her.	Disconnect, Trauma	Baseline stillness through most of trauma markers;
She is *crying or **distraught*** thinking about something.	Disconnect, Trauma	shallow breathing (freeze)
She *experiences some news, or she's thinking about something, or she got upset hearing something unpleasant. Hearing some bad news or having a big disappointment.* She puts	Disconnect Agency: action,	Even flow – breathing eases); tension moving away from face and upper body. After returning picture comes the biggest movement involving
her feet down and sits there for a little while and looks around. She's sad and has to		shoulders, upper back, neck, and head followed by sequential (left-right)
get up and *get over it.* In a	Disconnect	toe-tapping
public space so she	Deactivate	
gets up and she leaves.	Agency: action	

Terri's feelings of isolation and agitation are accompanied by freezing and stillness. We can also see how deactivating defenses combined with a description of the character's ability to move her body (put feet down, get up) is duplicated in Terri's corresponding release of tension and ease in breathing. She functionally shifts her attention away from her trauma.

The last three stimuli – Ambulance, Cemetery, and Corner – are the most intense and potentially activating scenes in the AAP (Buchheim et al., 2006). All three of Terri's stories reveal segregated trauma, and all demonstrate patterns of a constricted torso and shallow breathing. In Ambulance, described in the previous section, Terri snaps abruptly to attention mode to receive the stimulus but does not complete the reach. She fails to extend her arms fully. She holds her body still as she describes the child's horror and confusion. When she is given the Corner picture, her limbs remain contracted. The picture shakes in her hands as she finishes the AAP with the story of the frightened, terrorized, and ashamed self.[3]

Corner	Defense	Movement
		Keeps holding gaze at therapist;
A child is being *punished* for something,	Deactivate	looks away with
he's made to stand in a corner, and		
he's being **struck.** *He did something*	Trauma	abrupt bound
he wasn't supposed to do or didn't	Deactivate	and direct
follow instructions. He was *naughty.*	Disconnect	movement; picture shakes

He's *afraid,* and he's trying to keep from being struck again. He's protecting his body, and he's turning his head away, so he doesn't get hit straight in the face.	Trauma Agency: action	in hands from wrists, arms held Holds look at therapist longer;
Got his back up against a corner, so all he can do is try to protect his face. He's	Trauma	head movement uses horizontal
afraid. He's thinking, "here it comes again, I'll try to protect myself. *It really*	Trauma	plane for the first time
hurts. He's hitting me too hard." He has to stay there for – seems to be a long time. *He has to turn around and put his head to the corner.* And stand there and	Trauma	
stand there and *father the parent comes back – his mother or father, they let him leave the room.* He can turn around	Traumatic shame	
and go to his room and *do what he's supposed to do.*	Deactivate Agency: action, Deactivate	

Intervention

The brain excludes information from consciousness to mitigate being overwhelmed by the physical body. Bowlby (1980) defined this process as defensive exclusion. Neuroscience refers to the concept neurons, which consolidate an event's details and inter-relationship through a conceptual hierarchy (Quiroga, 2017). Thus "memory" may be thought of as a hierarchical process of selective forgetting rather than recording a perfectly ordered sequence of events for conscious recall (Quiroga, 2017). Attachment classifications are conceived as a *status.* This term indicates open to change; neuroplasticity is an integral layer of this fluid and associative construct. Science shows us that our memory is available for reorganizing conceptual associations through further learning (Calvo Tapia et al., 2020; Ison et al., 2015).

While episodic memory usually presents with missing details or patches of amnesia, implicit memory displays memories encoded before language development. These memories are encoded as a sensory recollection in the form of muscle tension, rhythms, use of space, and other kinesthetic cues. Slowing down a repetitive or dissociated gesture or posture often unearths emotions embedded in implicit memory, paving the way for future integration. In Terri's case, adding Sensorimotor Psychotherapy, a targeted somatic trauma protocol, to movement therapy disrupted the affect associated with traumatic memory and promoted self-regulation (Ogden et al., 2006).

Terri's reach and breathing through the AAP were habitually abrupt and contracted. The intervention for reach and breathing began by re-enacting the reach gesture, slowing it down gradually in small increments. It is common for physical sensations, emotions, and memories or thoughts to arise during this process. I asked her to stop when tension appeared in any part of her body or were activated and to slowly reverse the movement stopping at the point in space where the activation abated. In this way, she had control of her movements. When she felt the tension release, she resumed the movement forward until reach, grasp, pull, and release became a fluid phrase accompanied by deeper breathing and an expression of satisfaction.

During therapy, she described multiple memories of her father pressing down, gripping her shoulder while whispering a reminder not to touch or ask for anything as she exited the car during family shopping trips. It was not surprising then that she reported limited mobility and pain in one shoulder. Focusing attention on her shoulder blades, she explored the fluidity and range of her reach. For the first time, Terri noticed her habit of holding her breath when she reached. She became aware of the connection between holding her breath, the tightness she experienced in her back, and how her thoughts often stopped her from asking for help. This insight was critical for Terri. Like the characters in the AAP stories, Terri never asked (reached out) for help. Representational change of the attachment self requires fortifying connections to others and breaking through compulsive self-reliance and independence to ask for help. The body supports representational change through movement (posture and gesture), creating somatic awareness within the context of insight.

Failure to mourn: Clearing representational and somatic space for the present

According to Bowlby (1980), mourning involves reformulating the representational self. The first step in grieving requires individuals to "name" and "see" traumatic experiences from the past that shape their responses to people, relationships, and situations in the present. Mourning is complete, so to speak, when the self is freed from the fear of remembering to evaluate and reformulate the affect and details of trauma into a representational story that fits their current goals and aspirations. Terri, in her status of Failed Mourning, shut down this process; her self-narrative and body were held hostage. She was, in effect, frozen in space and time, holding on to the past.

The stillness of limbs and torso Teri showed in response to the most dysregulating AAP stimuli, Ambulance and Corner, revealed a strategy of immobilization that the Kestenberg Movement Profile refers to as "deep neutral flow" (Amighi et al., 2018). This perspective is consistent with Porges' (2011) polyvagal theory. This model categorizes a shutting down of the body's autonomic systems and use of muscle tone, either losing control or freezing, as the oldest phylogenetic response to a threat from which one cannot escape (Amighi et al., 2018). The notion that the muscular system possesses psychological functioning is also the centerpiece of an extensively documented Danish system of developmentally based healing for adults called Bodynamics (Marcher & Fich, 2010).

Terri's physical response to Ambulance evidenced immobility and maintaining low muscle tone. I addressed her response by bringing awareness of weight to the sit bones and limbs and working with her to feel the difference between the sensation of yield and collapse. This process enabled Terri to push and feel the support of her own body through connection to her spine. She stood and moved forward out of the freeze response by literally walking out of the room, transforming her trauma-induced immobility to a response of agency of self, the capacity to act. Terri explored the space, following her body's cues to move and breathe while conscious of emerging sensations, feelings, and thoughts. With this exploration, the embodied AAP narrative "came to life." Terri achieved closure by reframing "loss" as clearing space to then fill with her wisdom and creativity (permission to explore) and a reawakened awareness of her body.

Holding onto the past was evident in her somatic response to the Bed. While holding the Bed picture, she engaged in repetitive quick movements of release and grasp as she played with catching the picture with her hands. The principle of kinesthetic awareness became apparent when I asked her to experiment with mindful grasping and releasing of keys, eyeglasses, and other objects she constantly complained of losing. Recounting her experience of loss and letting go, Terri began to recall previously forgotten positive interactions with her father. She allowed herself to feel the part of her that missed him, eventually crying tears of recognition and grief for the first time since his death, beginning to process her Failed Mourning.

Three years later: Return to treatment

Three years later, during the COVID pandemic, Terri returned to treatment. She was reeling from the deaths of her long-time business partner and her mother within months of each other. I re-administered the AAP. Terri's attachment classification had changed from Dismissing, Failed Mourning to Preoccupied.

The follow-up AAP suggested that she had broken through her deactivating shield and had begun to grieve. Despite being a bit muddled (preoccupation created by cognitive disconnection), she was potentially on a path toward integration and earned security. Terri's new AAP showed several notable progress points in this direction. The only two stories evidencing residues of trauma were Window and Corner. This time in Window, Terri named the helplessness she felt but attributed it to conditions in the present (the COVID pandemic) rather than the past. She manages her trauma at the representational level with two forms of agency – the internalized secure base leading to the capacity to act. Her capacity to act involved a vision of connecting to her mother to ask for help.

As previously, Terri's Corner story was one of isolation and physical assault. It is the only story that evidenced remnants of a deactivating wall. However, Terri demonstrated how she now used deactivation and agentic self-protection to engage in the internalized secure base. She could now think about her parents' anger and her punishment rather than describing robotic compliance. Confronted with loss in Cemetery, Terri's story showed sentimental appreciation for a deceased loved one and a need to remember the past and communicate something to the deceased. She acknowledged that the character was grieving, but her story fell short of demonstrating that she had mourned her losses. Other stories suggested that she still struggled with expressing her attachment needs and anger and disappointment in relationships.

Conclusion

The foundation of the AAP's measurement of adult attachment status speaks directly to a developmental attachment model (George & West, 2012). Assessment reveals the representational status of the attachment system at any given time across the life span. Bowlby (1982) emphasized that the "working" element in the phrase "internal working model" involves processes that are open to updating and change.

This view crosses paths with the world of movement in Thelen and Smith's (1994) Dynamic Systems Theory of cognition and motor development, where the environment influences the individual. Laban (2011), Kestenberg (1885), and Lamb (2012) spoke of body, effort, shape, and space as elements that impact human movement and emotional states throughout the life span. Goldman (2004) observes that integrated movement's contribution to consciousness is that it must not only be noticed but actually felt. Cohen (2018) explores neurocellular patterns of development through movement based upon the principle that we do not discard our early development but build on it.

The AAP is an assessment tool and a navigation aid through the language of mental representation to the internal systems we cannot always express in words. The AAP's design creates a container for real-time viewing of the body's response to the activated attachment system. The lines of communication between mind and body that inform movement behavior extend beyond the brain and nervous system to include the musculoskeletal system, organs, glands, and the minutiae of intercellular function (Aposhyan, 1999). Including the body's contribution expands options and promotes understanding of the fundamental role of embodiment in assessing adult attachment.

Notes

1 Italics = defense
2 Italics = defense; bold = trauma; underline = capacity to act
3 Italics = defense; bold = trauma; underline = capacity to act

References

Ainsworth, M. D. S., Blehar, M., Waters, E., & Wall, S. (1978). *Patterns of attachment: A psychological study of the Strange Situation.* Erlbaum.

Amighi, J. K., Loman, S., & Sossin, K. M. (2018). *The meaning of movement: Embodied developmental, clinical, and cultural perspectives of the Kestenberg movement profile* (2nd ed). Routledge.

Aposhyan, S. (1999). *Natural intelligence: body-mind integration and human development.* Williams & Wilkins.

Bowlby, J. (1973). *Attachment and loss, Vol. 2. Separation: Anxiety and anger.* Basic Books.

Bowlby, J. (1980). *Attachment and loss, Vol. 3. Loss: Sadness and depression.* Basic Books.

Bowlby, J. (1982). *Attachment and loss, Vol. 1. Attachment.* Basic Books. (Original work published in 1969.)

Buchheim, A., Erk, S., George, C., Kaechele, H., Ruchsow, M., Spitzer, M., Kircher, T., & Walter, H. (2006). Measuring attachment representation in an fMRI environment: A pilot study. *Psychopathology, 39*(3), 144–152. https://doi.org/10.1159/000091800

Calvo Tapia, C., Tyukin, I., & Makarov, V. A. (2020). Universal principles justify the existence of concept cells. *Scientific Reports, 10*(1), 7889. https://doi.org/10.1038/s41598-020-64466-7

Cohen, B.B. (2018). Basic neurocellular patterns, exploring developmental movement. Burchfield Rose Publishers.

Frank, R., & La Barre, F. (2011). *The first year and the rest of your life: Movement, development, and psychotherapeutic change.* Routledge.

George, C., & West, M. (2012). *The adult attachment projective picture system: Attachment theory and assessment in adults.* Guilford Press.

Goldman, E. (2004). *As others see us: Body movement and the art of successful communication.* Routledge.

Ison, M. J., Quiroga, R. Q., & Fried, I (2015). Rapid encoding of new memories by individual neurons in the human brain. *Neuron, 87*(1), 220–230. https//doi.org/10.1016/j.neuron.2015.06.016

Kestenberg, J. S. (1995). *Sexuality, body movement, and the rhythms of development.* Jason Aronson.

Laban, R. (2011). *Choreutics.* L. Ullmann, (Ed.). Dance Books. (Original work published 1966).

Lamb, W. (2012). *A framework for understanding movement...My seven creative concepts.* Brechen Books.

Marcher, L., & Fich, S. (2010). *Body encyclopedia: A guide to the psychological functions of the muscular system.* North Atlantic Books.

Ogden, P., Minton, K., & Pain, C. (2006). *Trauma and the body: A sensorimotor approach to psychotherapy.* W. W. Norton.

Quiroga, R. Q. (2017). *The forgetting machine*. BenBella Books.

Shafir, T. B. (2015). Bridging the trauma-adult attachment connection through somatic movement. *Body, Movement and Dance in Psychotherapy, 10*(4), 243–255. https://doi.org/10.1080/17432979.2015.1067256

Shafir, T. B. (2019). An examination of the relationship between somatic movement patterns and adult attachment status. [Unpublished doctoral dissertation]. International University of Professional Studies, Maui, Hawaii.

Thelen, E., & Smith, L. B. (1994). *A dynamic systems approach to the development of cognition and action*. MIT Press.

Tsachor, R. P., & Shafir, T. (2017). A somatic movement approach to fostering emotional resiliency through Laban movement analysis. *Frontiers of Human Neuroscience,* https://doi.org/10.3389/fnhum.2017.00410

10 Using the Adult Attachment Projective Picture System in a transdiagnostic approach during psychoanalytic treatment

Therapy and neurophysiological outcomes

Anna Buchheim

Bowlby's (1988) proposals for attachment-informed psychotherapy are increasingly relevant today and have been incorporated into the practices of many psychotherapists using a relational approach (e.g., Bateman & Fonagy, 2006; Holmes, 2001). He formulated five attachment-based therapeutic tasks: (1) therapist as a secure base for self-exploration, (2) reflection of inner working models in present relationships, (3) examination of the therapeutic relationship, (4) genesis of inner working models in the attachment representations of the parents, and (5) reality check of the "old" inner working models for appropriateness. This chapter examines the application of the Adult Attachment Projective Picture System (AAP) in the context of these goals during psychoanalytic treatment. The chapter first describes the common ground of attachment and psychoanalysis, focusing on the valuable contribution of attachment theory to psychotherapy, and then introduces a neuropsychoanalytic single case study on a depressive patient with oscillating shifts of mood. We used various assessments to show the interplay of attachment, psychoanalysis, and neuroimaging.

Common ground of attachment theory and psychoanalysis

Attachment theory concepts such as the secure base and internal working models are suitable for evaluating individuals' ability to flexibly integrate positive and negative aspects of the self and significant others. One primary goal of psychotherapy is to change or reorganize dysfunctional aspects of the self and others (Davila & Levy, 2006). Moreover, the focus of many psychodynamic approaches is on improving self- and relationship-regulation and the ability to recognize, understand, and think about one's own internal processes and those of significant others.

DOI: 10.4324/9781003215431-13

This approach constitutes a common ground of attachment theory and psychoanalysis.

Results from psychodynamic studies using attachment measures

Current psychodynamic psychotherapy studies using attachment measures to evaluate their effects demonstrate the capacity for representational change from Unresolved to Secure or organized attachment representations and improved mentalizing ability (Buchheim et al., 2017, 2018; Fischer-Kern et al., 2015; Levy et al., 2006). Thus, attachment measures can contribute significantly to the evidence of a positive outcome of the therapeutic process. Recent transdiagnostic approaches suggest the importance of identifying factors and processes related to risk, protection, and maintenance implicated in mental health problems by assessing biological, socioenvironmental, and psychological characteristics (Dalgleish et al., 2020).

Accordingly, recent psychotherapy studies have combined attachment and neuroscience measures to map changes in neural activation (e.g., in the amygdala or hippocampus areas) during psychodynamic psychotherapy to verify mental change (Buchheim et al., 2012, 2013, 2018). In these studies, the AAP was used for developing fMRI paradigms to demonstrate neural changes during therapy when individuals are presented with personalized attachment material.

The activation of the attachment system during psychotherapy is inevitable, given its intimate and relational nature. These qualities of psychotherapy highlight the importance of considering attachment-related themes and processes to understand better the therapeutic relationship and process (Dozier & Brady, 2004). Knowledge of attachment patterns can be constructive for therapists when working in the here and now to confront patients with their distorted representations of self and significant others (Buchheim et al., 2017; Levy et al., 2006).

Neuropsychoanalytic study

Psychoanalysis has a long tradition of using single case studies to evaluate clinical material and the therapy process (Kächele et al., 2006). Single-case studies have also been presented in the field of neuroscientific application (Schiepek et al., 2009).

For the first time, this author and her colleagues (2013) conducted a single-case design study to empirically examine process and change during psychoanalytic psychotherapy with a dysthymic patient. The study used repetitive examinations on various methodological assessments such as self-report, neuroimaging, and projective and shed light on the interaction of these assessments. The Adult Attachment Projective

Picture System (AAP, George & West, 2012) was used to assess attachment-related defense processes and the neurophysiological experimental procedure. The analyst's subjective assessment of the therapy sessions was also documented, and the Psychotherapy Q-Set was used to evaluate objectively 12 of the transcribed sessions (Jones, 2000). Lastly, the study considered the neurophysiological effects of attachment activation using the AAP stimuli by using 12 fMRI measurements (Buchheim et al., 2012).

This study was the first time the AAP had been used to evaluate attachment-related defensive processes to validate the psychodynamics and transference processes of a patient (see Buchheim et al., 2013 for a complete description of the study), as well as to measure change in the attachment representation after one year of treatment. The treatment was designed as a low-frequency long-term analytic therapy. The observation period was 12 months, and data were collected at regular intervals every four weeks. The AAP was not used to plan the main goals of the therapy. Instead, it was used during a critical phase of treatment to objectify the patient's clinical features and evaluate the outcome. It was also used to systematically validate the therapist's subjective interpretation of the patient's problems.

Lore: A single case study

Lore is a 42-year-old woman with doctoral-level education who was struggling with oscillating affective states. Upon waking, she knew whether that day would be an "easy" or a "heavy" day (i.e., difficult) since she was well familiar with her past shifting mood states. Her mood on heavy days prevented her from concentrating and working successfully. She felt depressed and was unable to think. On these days, Lore isolated herself by withdrawing from relationships and worked hard to hide her emotional vulnerability. On the "easy" days, Lore was productive and engaged. Lore's stagnant depression sometimes shifted to manic states, and her fragile and vulnerable sense of self and others were central aspects of the psychoanalytic treatment during this stage of therapy.

The psychoanalyst considered two deaths to be essential contributors to Lore's symptoms. One was the loss of her mother when she was 30 years old. One of the lingering overarching feelings she experienced was guilt. She felt guilty because she could not call the emergency doctor in enough time to save her mother. The second loss coincided with the birth of her first child and involved the tragic death of a colleague. Again, Lore felt guilty because she could not reach her colleague in enough time to help her. The analyst also considered Lore's current long-term partnership to contribute to her emotional difficulties. Lore described this relationship as distant and competitive, with feelings of rivalry and envy. She and her partner were in constant, seemingly unsolvable conflict, and Lore repeatedly considered separating.

The AAP was used at mid-treatment to gain a deeper understanding of Lore's attachment-related defenses in both the alone and dyadic stories and evaluate for potential unresolved issues (see Chapter 1). Lore's AAP classification was Unresolved for attachment trauma, which is not surprising given her history of loss, feelings of guilt, and conflictual relationships. The dysregulation that determined her unresolved status emerged in response to the Cemetery picture. The Cemetry scene is conceived as confronting the speaker with a past relationship. The dysregulated element of her Cemetery story is shown here[1]:

A man at the grave, that is not a fresh grave, it is long ago. It is the loss. *I'm not sure right now if the person who died was*	Disconnect
his wife or his father... where you come back you also relate to and don't often get there, so physical direction... *It's a*	Trauma
dialogue with, yeah, four eyes see more than two.	

This story ends with the living engaged in a dialogue with the deceased person. The fact that the deceased is portrayed as engaged in reciprocal conversation demonstrates the traumatic quality of this representational encounter. Lore's continued immersion in her past becomes perceptible, and the statement that "four eyes see more than two" connotes a spectral, ghostly quality from which she does not recover (i.e., the spectral material remains uncontained). Lore's Unresolved status shows that she lives in a chronic state of mourning that she is unable to contain when flooded by memories of the past. (see Chapter 4).

In addition to Cemetery, two of Lore's other alone stories were central in formulating her case. She told the following story to Bench[2]:

A young woman who is alone, *thinking*, I also see a little bit, so the question of loneliness, of	Agency: internalized secure base,
abandonment, but also so the self-contained, that	Trauma
perhaps they also want to withdraw, to *withdraw to*	
themselves to think. So this, yes, there is something	Agency: internalized
self-contained about it. Oh, I think that when she	secure base
has been completely with herself, she will then get up	Agency: action
and look forward and go further. Whether she will	
overcome or bypass the *wall remains the question.*	Disconnected trauma

The Bench narrative demonstrated how Lore's integration (internalized secure base) leads to future action (get up) after feeling abandoned and isolated. The narrative also shows Lore's repetitive mode of integration when alone requires disconnecting by withdrawing, remaining closed in, and being entirely with oneself rather than reaching out to others, such as attachment figures or friends. Even acknowledging her resources for agency, Lore continues to question her regulatory effectiveness.

She told the following story to Corner[3]:

So, this *distance*, the head is turned away, for me it	Deactivate
means, I don't know if it has something to do with	
shame or being ashamed or guilt, being conscious of	Disconnected shame
guilt, not wanting to bring accusations upon oneself,	
not wanting to have them. So, like that, yes, he had	Deactivate
a mission and *had not fulfilled it.* The question is, is	Deactivate
he *frightened, afraid* of the other. I don't think he's	Segregated system
afraid of punishment, but rather he realizes his own	Disconnect →
guilt and even wants to *push away his own guilt.* The	Deactivate
friend who helped him with the *job* comes, and he	Deactivate
takes him by the hands and then hugs him.	

In this narrative, we see that Lore's attachment-relevant resources are represented by connection to and external help from a friend, which help regulate her when frightened. This description suggests that Lore has an internal idea of managing attachment-relevant situations that are anxiety-provoking (lurking disconnected shame, guilt) through help from a close person. The narrative also shows that Lore does not view the self as having any agency when severely distressed, contrary to Bench. Instead, a person must notice her distress and come and help her. Lore is not inclined to seek help proactively. We also see that the close person from whom she receives help is not a stronger and wiser attachment figure (i.e., parent) but a friend. This story tells us that when Lore's attachment system is highly activated, her attention shifts to care provided by individuals in her peer system (a friend) instead of the attachment system (a caregiver). The story elements also reveal Lore's need to deactivate and neutralize negative self-evaluation and accusations defensively; she consciously rejects the negative affect and shame that is activated before the connection to a friend is described.

Lore's internal working model when attachment figures are accessible (dyadic pictures) showed no expectations for sensitive care (synchrony) and demonstrated even more pronounced defensive deactivation (distancing, rejection) than representations of the alone self. Her dyadic responses were punctuated with lengthy mental interruptions (pauses) in the narrative and disconnection evidenced by confusion about attachment situations. Attachment figures, however, are portrayed as potentially available to help her manage attachment distress. Lore's Departure story was an exception[4]:

That's the picture of setting off on the journey, where *you*	
don't really know if both want the journey or was it initiated	Disconnect
by him {pause} and there's a certain *reserve* on the part of	
his partner. But both have their hands in their pockets, not	
wanting to communicate with each other. The *distance* is	Deactivate
big. {pause} Could be a conversation, but it is certainly not a	
completely loving conversation, rather a bit *silent between the*	Deactivate
two, a departure to something new with a certain *distance.*	Deactivate

Yes, but with her insecurity: *Do I want this, do I want to go further, drive with him?* (What might happen next?) A big difficult now. {pause} of course, guided by the long experience in this relationship, there is no rapprochement, no understanding, and he says, "everyone gets on this train by himself." {pause} A journey into the *unknown*.	Disconnect Disconnect

This story echoes Lore's core themes: her impaired ability to think and speak (long pause, silences) and withdrawal. When she is depressed, she cannot concentrate and withdraws. She cannot work. Her disconnection is related to her symptoms of depression (West & George, 2002). The narrative also depicts her relationship closeness-distance problems. The relationship is depicted by silence. The characters are emotionally independent and separate even though they physically travel together. Lacking feelings of intimate togetherness and mutual enjoyment, Lore remains confused as to how this arrangement of mutual independence will work out in the end.

Psychodynamics and neural correlates of the psychoanalytic treatment

Lore was treated using standard long-term psychoanalysis with two face-to-face sessions per week. Interpretive interventions aimed to enhance her insight into the repetitive conflicts sustaining her problems were used. They engaged in supportive interventions aimed to strengthen abilities that were not sufficiently developed or temporarily inaccessible due to acute distress (e.g., traumatic events).

The AAP was administered at the beginning of treatment and one year later to assess potential changes in Lore's coping strategies and ability to manage attachment distress. Lore also completed several fMRI scans throughout this period. Twelve psychoanalytic sessions were tape-recorded and evaluated using the Psychotherapy Process Q-Sort (PQS, Jones, 2000) by two independent, blind raters with established satisfactory results inter-rater reliability (Labek, 2011).

The therapist also described their subjective impressions of Lore's problems during the analysis. The analyst documented the following themes as central to understanding Lore's psychodynamics:

> In the depressive patient, there was a connection of the symptomatology with culpable processing of losses and strong fears and mourning processes arising from this. On the difficult (heavy) days, there was a massive inhibition of thinking and an inability to name thoughts and feelings during these hours. A deeply anchored lack of self-esteem accompanied difficult days. While the patient sank into silence on heavy days, she talked expansively and showed extroversion on the light days.

Table 10.1 shows a comprehensive comparison between Lore's AAP and the psychoanalyst's evaluations.

The PQS is a 100-item Q-Sort measure used in psychotherapy research to assess individual therapy sessions by evaluating the attitude, behavior, and experience of the patient and therapist and their interaction. The PQS describes and classifies the therapy process in a standardized format (Jones, 2000; Labek, 2011). The PQS items were subjected to a principal component analysis to capture the essential aspects of the analyst's description of the clinical situation. In this way, it was possible to evaluate blind-rated

Table 10.1 Lore's Psychodynamic Characteristics, PQS Items, and AAP Evaluation

Patient's Psychodynamic Characteristics	*Characteristic PQS-Items Evaluated in 12 Therapy Sessions*	*AAP Evaluation at the Beginning of Treatment*
Massive inhibition of thinking and inability to name thoughts and feelings	"Patient has difficulty starting the lesson" (Item 25)	In the AAP Picture *"Departure"* long pauses in the narrative and an impaired ability to talk about thoughts and feelings in the relationship
While the patient talks expansively on "easy" days, she sinks silently into herself on "hard" days	"There is silence during the lessons" (*Item 12*)	In the AAP Picture *"Bench"* withdrawal, being completely with oneself In the AAP Picture *"Departure"* long pauses in the narrative
Guilty processing of losses and resulting strong fears and mourning processes	"Patient is anxious or tense vs. calm and relaxed" (Item 7)	In the AAP picture *"Cemetery"* ghostly quality, which could be related to fearful events and indicates a blurring of the boundaries between the living and the dead. Indication of unprocessed grief In the AAP picture *"Corner"* defense markers of deactivation, which are represented here in form of punishment, accusation, as well as negative evaluation of the person in the story including shame
Massive inhibition of thinking and inability to name thoughts and feelings	"Patient does not initiate topics or elaborate on topics" (*Item 15*)	See above for AAP picture *"Departure"*
Strong fears and mourning processes	"Patient is anxious or worried about her dependence on the therapist vs. comfortable with dependence or wants dependence" (*Item 8*)	See above for AAP pictures *"Cemetery"* and *"Corner"*

therapy sessions with an objective and validated method. Lore's PQS analysis is also shown in Table 10.1. The pattern showed that this objective instrument could reliably characterize the sessions (hard and light).

In the analyst's sessions rated as light, Lore was engaged with relationship issues in the therapeutic dyad and expressed more emotion. The sessions rated as hard were characterized by silence, anxiety, tension, withdrawal, and distancing. Lore's AAP showed that at times she had agency for action and mental resources (internalized secure base), which were probably evidenced in the light sessions. The AAP also showed unprocessed mourning and deactivation defenses associated with the feelings of fear, punishment, guilt, shame, withdrawal into herself, and impaired emotionality. These were qualities that Lore most likely exhibited during the hard sessions.

An important research question in the present case, and the study as a whole, was whether neuroimaging data obtained could corroborate this difference in mental and emotional states evidenced during the light and hard sessions. To answer this question, Lore participated in an fMRI attachment paradigm developed by the author and her colleagues that was tailor-made for each patient and consisted of 12 administrations over the treatment year (Buchheim et al., 2013). In this paradigm, Lore was presented with core sentences extracted from her AAP narratives (see Figure 10.1) and standard neutral sentences serving as controls. The interaction effect of session quality assessed by the analyst (light or hard) and personal relevance of the stimulus material (core AAP sentences) was calculated.

The fMRI analysis of Lore's scans showed significant activation in the posterior cingulate cortex during the hard sessions over time. Previous

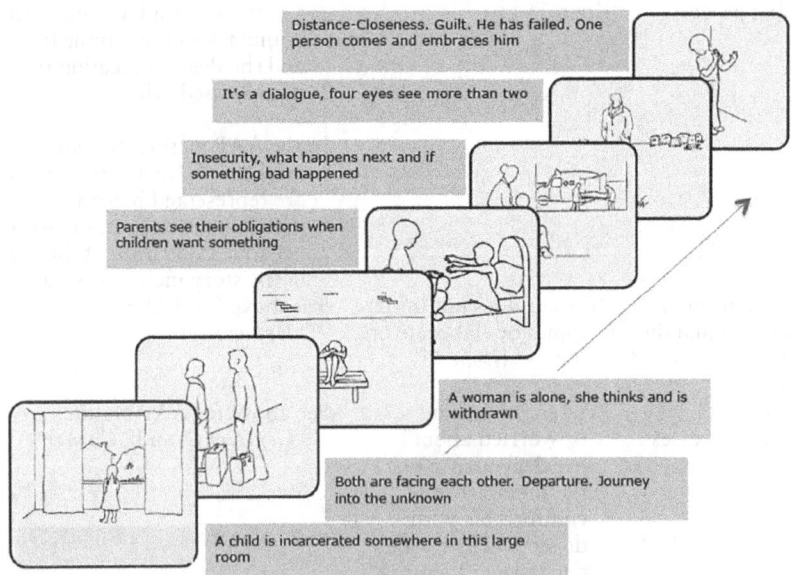

Figure 10.1 Personalized fMRI-AAP paradigm based on Buchheim et al. (2012).

fMRI studies reported that the posterior cingulate cortex is modulated when participants are asked to distance themselves from negative topics (e.g., social interactions) (Koenigsberg et al., 2010) or when they were emotionally dysregulated (Doering et al., 2012). This activation in Lore's scans was interpreted as an indication of emotional self-distancing processes observed in her AAP narratives. In essence, her defense formations on hard days (silence, inhibition) were evident on a neuronal level. Lore's fMRI evaluation confirmed stable patterns that corresponded with the analyst's clinical impression, the PQS-analysis, and the AAP assessment.

Clinical implications

The Buchheim et al. (2013) study attempted to objectify a clinical description of the psychoanalytic process using three empirical instruments to shed a more profound light on patients' defensive structures during the treatment phase. The aim was to investigate the influence of fluctuating mental states and their effect on the therapeutic interaction on a clinical, attachment, and neural level.

For Lore, the results helped the psychoanalyst gain a deeper understanding of the persistently fluctuating dynamic of the transference relationship mirrored by her experiences of los. This information helped the therapist cope with diverse negative counter-transference feelings (helplessness, hope, anger). Lore felt she had failed to prevent the unexpected deaths. For a particular time during the treatment, the analyst and the patient failed to find ways to help her regulate and stabilize her emotional instability and unpredictable mood shifts. During this phase of treatment, Lore's depressive symptoms did not change significantly. This lack of change was problematic for the therapist. However, Lore's AAP after one year of treatment demonstrated a vital shift. Her attachment classification changed from Unresolved to Dismissing. The classification change was a valuable indicator of Lore's progress for the therapist. Her dysregulated-unresolved story to Cemetery changed after one year of treatment into a regulated-organized narrative characterized by metacognition and the internalized secure base that integrated the resolution process associated with mourning. Her therapist's notes also described this qualitative shift. Here is the follow-up Cemetery story[5]:

The person comes to the grave of his father or another beloved person, and he has remained in an *inner dialogue* with him. Even if one does not love these rituals like cemetery, they have a function, a reactivation of memories can bring closeness. On the	Metacognitive monitoring
one hand, he *thinks*, it's a pit, it's sad, that you're not here anymore, that you left so early, so surprisingly, so early, but you gave us a lot, and we're actually *big*	Agency: internalized secure base
and *strong* to keep you inside and to cope with it.	Deactivate

This follow-up narrative suggests that the treatment was successful in helping Lore overcome the helplessness she experienced in response to her significant losses. Her current attachment representation shows that she monitors her affect and thoughts (metacognitive monitoring). It also shows the integrative power of the internalized secure base in mourning. She realized that the relationship with the beloved person was valued (you gave us a lot). Compare this story with the traumatic haunting evidenced in the unresolved and impersonal version of Cemetery she told prior to therapy (It is the loss. I'm not sure right now if the person who died was his wife or father). In addition to the resolution of mourning, Lore's follow-up AAP showed how effective deactivation defenses and her view that others eliminated stories about a frightened self. Deactivation is a normalizing defense. As such, we would expect that Lore's need for distance and independence in relationships could give way to functional togetherness, that is, to "just be" with friends and partners without needing to construct walls.

Like Bowlby's (1988) suggestions for therapeutic goals, the analyst helped Lore cope with traumatic pain and rework her representation of self and others within the therapeutic relationship. One major focus of the treatment was to increase Lore's ability to react in a timely way to future distressing events, like illness or death, to help her process them in a more controlled and integrated way. This goal was supported by Lore's demonstration of metacognitive thinking about attachment events. Another aim was to improve her capacity to differentiate between reality and fantasy by enhancing self-reflection, which was successfully evidenced by Lore's internalized secure base in Cemetery. We may conclude that, according to Bowlby, the analyst served as a secure base for self-exploration and structural change. Lore gained enhanced access and the ability to think about her attachment experiences in an integrated way. Most importantly, with the help of her analyst, she was able to grieve her losses. Lore's resolution of her pathological mourning opens the door to potential new growth, deepened connection with self and others, and emotional stability.

Notes

1 Italics = defenses; bold = trauma
2 Italics = defenses; bold = trauma; underline = capacity to act
3 Italics = defenses
4 Italics = defenses
5 Italics = defenses

References

Bateman, A. W., & Fonagy, P. (2006). *Mentalization-based treatment for borderline personality disorder: A practical guide.* Oxford University Press.

Bowlby, J. (1988). *A secure base*. Basic Books.

Buchheim, A., Hörz-Sagstetter, S., Döring, S., Rentrop, M., Schuster, P., Buchheim, P., Pokorny, D., & Fischer-Kern, M. (2017). Change of unresolved attachment in borderline personality disorder: RCT Study of transference-focused psychotherapy. *Psychotherapy and Psychosomatics, 86*(5), 314–316. https://doi.org/10.1159/000460257

Buchheim, A., Labek, K., Taubner, S., Kessler, H., Pokorny, D., Kächele, H., Cierpka, M., Roth, G., Pogarell, O., & Karch, S. (2018). Modulation of gamma band activity and late positive potential in patients with chronic depression after psychodynamic psychotherapy. *Psychotherapy and Psychosomatics, 87*(4), 252–254. https://doi.org/10.1159/000488090

Buchheim, A., Labek, K., Walter, S., & Viviani, R. (2013). A clinical case study of a psychoanalytic psychotherapy monitored with functional neuro-imaging. *Frontiers in Human Neuroscience*, https://doi.org/10.3389/fnhum.2013.00677

Buchheim, A., Viviani, R., Kessler, H., Kächele, H., Cierpka, M., Roth, G., George, C., Kernberg, O. F., Bruns, G., & Taubner, S. (2012). Changes in prefrontal-limbic function in major depression after 15 months of long-term psychotherapy. *PLoS One, 7*(3), 1–8. https://doi.org/10.1371/journal.pone.0033745

Dalgleish, T., Black, M., Johnston, D., & Bevan, A. (2020). Transdiagnostic approaches to mental health problems: Current status and future directions. *Journal of Consulting and Clinical Psychology, 88*(3), 179–195. http://doi.org/10.1037/ccp0000482

Davila, J., & Levy, K. N. (2006): Introduction to the special section on attachment theory and psychotherapy. *Journal of Consulting and Clinical Psychology, 74*(6), 989–993. https://doi.org/10.1037/0022–006X.74.6.989.

Doering, S., Enzi, B., Faber, C., Hinrichs, J., Bahmer, J., & Northoff, G. (2012). Personality functioning and the cortical midline structures: An exploratory fMRI study. *PLoS One, 7*(11), 1–8. https://doi.org/10.1371/journal.pone.0049956

Dozier, M., & Bates, B. C. (2004). Attachment state of mind and the treatment relationship. In L. Atkinson & S. Goldberg (Eds.), *Attachment issues in psychopathology and intervention* (pp. 167–180). Erlbaum.

Fischer-Kern, M., Doering, S., Taubner, S., Hörz-Sagstetter, S., Buchheim, P., Rentrop, M., Schuster, P., & Buchheim, A. (2015). Transference-focused psychotherapy for borderline personality disorder: Change in reflective function. *British Journal of Psychiatry, 207*(2), 173–174. https://doi.org/10.1192/bjp.bp.113.143842.

George, C., & West, M. (2012). *The adult attachment projective picture system*. Guilford Press.

Holmes, J. (2001). *The search for the secure base: Attachment theory and psychotherapy*. Routledge.

Jones, E. E. (2000). *Therapeutic action: A guide to psychoanalytic therapy*. Jason Aronson.

Kächele, H., Albani, C., Buchheim, A., Hölzer, M., Hohage, R., Mergenthaler, E., Jiménez, J. P., Leuzinger-Bohleber, M., Neudert-Dreyer, L., & Pokorny, D. (2006).The German specimen case Amalia X: Empirical studies. *International Journal of Psychoanalysis, 87*(3), 1–18. https://doi.org/10.1516/17NN-M9HJ-U25A-YUU5

Koenigsberg, H. W., Fan, J., Ochsner, K. N., Liu, X., Guise, K., Pizzarello, S., Dorantes, C., Tecuta, L., Guerreri, S., Goodman, M., New, A., Flory, J., & Siever, L. J. (2010). Neural correlates of using distancing to regulate emotional responses to social situations. *Neuropsychologia, 48*(6), 813–1822. https://doi.org/10.1016/j.neuropsychologia.2010.03.002

Labek, K. (2011). Psychoanalytische Psychotherapieforschung: Auswertung eines Einzelfalls einer depressiven Patientin mit dem *Psychotherapie Prozess Q-Set* [Unpublished manuscript]. Univerity of Innsbruck, Austria.

Levy, K. N., Meehan, K. B., Kelly, K. M., Reynoso, J. S., Weber, M., Clarkin, J. F., & Kernberg, O. F. (2006). Change in attachment patterns and reflective function in a randomized control trial of transference-focused psychotherapy for borderline personality disorder. *Journal of Consulting and Clinical Psychology, 74*(6), 1027–1040. https://doi.org/10.1037/0022-006X.74.6.1027

Schiepek, G., Tominschek, I., Karch, S., Lutz, J., Mulert, C., Meindl, T., & Pogarell, O. (2009). A controlled single case study with repeated fMRI measures during the treatment of a patient with obsessive-compulsive disorder: Testing the nonlinear dynamics approach to psychotherapy. *The World Journal of Biological Psychiatry, 10*(4), 658–668. https://doi.org/10.1080/15622970802311829

West, M., & George, C. (2002). Attachment and dysthymia: The contributions of preoccupied attachment and agency of self to depression in women. *Attachment and Human Development, 4*(3), 278–293. https://doi.org/10.1080/14616739900134201

11 Confusion, fear, and loss

Clinical applications of the AAP with people with intellectual disabilities

Deanna Gallichan, Nancy Poulter, Alex Clark, and Kate Stoneman

This chapter uses two clinical cases to demonstrate the use of the Adult Attachment Projective Picture System (AAP) with people with intellectual disabilities. Intellectual disability (ID) is an internationally recognized term defined by the World Health Organization as:

> a significantly reduced ability to understand new or complex information and to learn and apply new skills (impaired intelligence). This results in a reduced ability to cope independently (impaired social functioning), and begins before adulthood, with a lasting effect on development (WHO Europe).

Intellectual disabilities can be associated with genetic conditions such as Down's syndrome, fragile X or DiGeorge syndrome, and neurodevelopmental conditions, such as autism and cerebral palsy. Individuals with ID also frequently have associated health problems and other disabilities (e.g., physical or sensory disabilities). The WHO's definition also includes developmental delays that are due to environmental or social factors, such as neglect or institutionalization in early childhood.

People with ID are as unique and variable as typically developing individuals. People with milder ID may be able to communicate well, work, live independently, and parent a child. At the other end of the spectrum, individuals with more severe ID may be minimally verbal or even non-verbal and require round the clock care.

Historically, clinical interventions for people with ID focused on observable behavior and interactions with their environment, most notably through applied behavioral analysis. In the 1990s, psychotherapists began to write about the internal world of their patients with ID, focusing on relationships, loss, and trauma (e.g., Sinason, 1992). Researchers began to focus on attachment theory around the turn of the century, initially focusing on children. A meta-analysis by Rutgers et al. (2004) demonstrated that attachment insecurity was more likely in children with autism who had lower levels of mental development

DOI: 10.4324/9781003215431-14

than in children with autism who had normal intelligence. They proposed that lower mental development, synonymous with ID, impacted the development of internal working models of attachment. Schuengel and Janssen (2006) suggested that differences in communication and signaling within attachment-caregiving dyads could challenge the development of attachment relationships for people with ID. They proposed that the need for professional caregivers into adulthood could impede the development of autonomy in this population, and therefore threaten the development of attachment security. People with ID are also at high risk for abuse across the life span (Horner-Johnson & Drum, 2006), experiences shown to undermine the development of a secure internal working model of attachment (Lyons-Ruth & Jacobwitz, 2016). In the UK, there is now professional guidance on incorporating attachment theory into clinical work for people with ID (British Psychological Society, 2016) and a dedicated volume on this topic (Fletcher et al., 2016).

Although attachment theory is now more prominent in clinical work with people with ID, further work is necessary to understand how ID impacts the development of internal working models of attachment. For many years, issues of measurement impeded progress in this area, but the AAP (George & West, 2012) has offered a solution to this impasse. The AAP is to date the only direct developmental measure of adult attachment that has demonstrated conceptual validity and inter-rater reliability in people with ID. The use of the AAP in this population was first described in Gallichan and George (2014), where a description of minor modifications to the procedure was followed by a case series linking clinical information to the AAP analysis. Gallichan and George (2018) went on to show that the AAP had good inter-rater reliability (80%) and face validity across a small sample of 20 individuals with ID. Most participants ($n = 12$) were classified as Unresolved. The high rates of attachment trauma in this sample were examined further in Gallichan and George (2016) by exploring links between themes of bullying and feelings of helplessness or terror.

These findings were replicated and extended by Bateman et al. (2020) who compared AAP classifications between a clinical and a non-clinical group in a sample of 24 individuals with ID. This study found similarly high rates of Unresolved attachment classifications and attachment trauma across the sample ($n = 16$), with no discernible difference between the clinical and non-clinical groups. This work provides further evidence that people with ID are at risk not only of attachment insecurity but also dysregulation associated with attachment trauma.

The two cases in this chapter illustrate how the AAP elucidated key features of the individual's internal working models of attachment, which supported a reformulation away from a behavioral perspective and toward a more attachment-oriented understanding of the clients' underlying emotional distress.

The first case, "Emma," illustrates many of the key features present in clinical work with adults with ID. The second case, "Grace," provides the first clinical description of the use of the AAP with an adolescent with ID. Both cases were referred to multidisciplinary teams run by the National Health Service in the UK. These teams offer specialist assessment and intervention to people with intellectual disabilities living in the community and are typically comprised of specialist nurses, occupational therapists, speech and language therapists, physiotherapists, psychiatrists, clinical psychologists, and other support staff. Teams work with the individual themselves, and their surrounding support network such as their families, professional caregivers, and in the case of children, school staff. Emma was referred to a team specializing in working with adults with ID, whereas Grace was referred to an ID specialist team working under the umbrella of Child and Adolescent Mental Health Services (CAMHS). Both cases were assessed using the adapted AAP protocol for people with ID as described by Gallichan and George (2014).

Emma

Emma, aged 51, was referred for help with distressed behavior that was thought to be triggered by relationship difficulties with her support workers. Emma lived in an apartment within a supported living complex with onsite staff. She received 21 hours of one-to-one support a week to help her with daily living skills, accessing the community, and emotional support. At the time of the referral, Emma said she was happy in her flat despite the long-standing difficulties in her relationships with support staff.

Initial assessments included a risk assessment, mental health screen, and clinical interviews with Emma's support workers, which included reviewing their behavior plans. The support workers described Emma as having an "explosive temper" and "mood swings." They reported that Emma swore, screamed, shouted, used aggressive hand gestures, threatened to harm others, slammed doors, and pushed past people. They also reported Emma became angry when she was asked to do something she did not want to do (including personal care, shopping, and cleaning the home).

Before the coronavirus pandemic, Emma had been attending an activity center for adults with ID. There, she was reported to be kind, sociable, and considerate. She had several friends and liked to offer help to others. Emma managed the coronavirus restrictions well, enjoying activities in her home when the activity center was closed.

Background

Emma was raised by her mother and was the middle child of three daughters. Her developmental milestones were delayed, and she transferred to a school for children with special educational needs when she was 7. There was not much information about her relationships with her family. For example, her father was absent for most of Emma's life but the reasons for this were not known. Emma was asked about memories of her early life, but she shared very little, often just stating "I don't know" or saying nothing at all. She mentioned enjoying holidays with her mother but did not elaborate further.

After leaving school, Emma remained living at home, but this quite quickly became challenging for Emma's mother. There were reports of aggression toward others in public and toward her mother at home from around the age of 19. At 26, Emma moved out of the family home to a placement with support staff, where she was able to have regular contact and visits with her mother. Emma then had a long series of short-lived supported living placements, which broke down in a repeating pattern. Support workers experienced Emma as "aggressive and controlling" and described her as appearing "jealous" of any attention shown to her peers, which led to her "manipulating" situations to draw the attention back to her. Attempts to manage these behaviors included reducing her support hours, but the difficulties would intensify, leading to staff refusing to work with her, ultimately meaning that Emma had to move on to a new home and new support team. These frequent moves made it very difficult to understand what Emma was experiencing, and it was hypothesized that this may have perpetuated her difficulties relating to new workers.

When Emma was 45, her mother passed away, and at the point of her referral six years later, Emma continued to become very emotional when talking about her mother's death. Emma refused contact with her siblings or other family members, but it was not clear why relationships had broken down.

In addition to multiple moves, there were several safeguarding[1] concerns over the years. These included Emma allowing a stranger posing as a gas engineer into her flat, a peer assault, an allegation of sexual assault, and an investigation into "controlling and abusive" care at her placement eight years before the referral. The latter led to the placement closing.

The long-standing and relational nature of Emma's difficulties led to an initial hypothesis that she may have an insecure internal working model of attachment. The AAP was offered to explore this further and aid the clinical formulation and intervention plan.

AAP assessment, classification, and analysis

Emma's communication profile was consulted before offering the AAP. A Speech and Language Therapist had assessed Emma as being able to understand simple instructions at a three key-word level,[2] make choices from two to three options, and express herself using short basic sentences. This suggested that Emma would be able to respond to the AAP and understand the instructions and prompts.

Emma agreed to complete the AAP, and encouragement was provided as appropriate to maintain her engagement without violating the AAP administration protocol. Emma's responses to the AAP probes generally consisted of a short description of the picture (e.g., "lady looking out" for Window), followed by "I don't know," and a feeling state (e.g., "angry" or "sad"). Initially, these sparse responses were thought to be an artifact of Emma's ID, but this idea was not congruent with her communication skills. The AAP was coded by a reliable judge who was blind to Emma's clinical detail and a master judge. They determined that Emma was able to provide some basic descriptions and feeling states. As such, Emma's story responses were sparse but codable. Emma depicted characters as very alone and neither engaging in functional action nor as having the capacity to think about problems and distress; they were left confused, angry, and sad. She was classified as Preoccupied. A detailed analysis of the content and defensive processes coding enabled us to develop a successful case formulation and intervention plan. We will use Emma's case to explore how sparse responses to the AAP, which can be common for people with ID, can reveal more than meets the eye.

Emma's response to Bench was typical of her AAP transcript[3]: Bench depicts a character alone, conceived to represent the projected self as being alone and distressed (George & West, 2012). Emma's disconnection was evidenced by the Bench character described as confused and

Hands together and head down (What happened before?) *I don't know.* (What do you think she is thinking or feeling?) *Angry.* (What is she thinking?). *I don't know.* (What happens next?). *I don't know.*	Disconnect Disconnect Disconnect

angry. She did not describe any agency or other resources from which to draw to address this discomfort. Emma became confused regarding why the character might be feeling this way or how the character might manage this anger. It is typical for individuals in a disconnected state of mind, as Emma is, to demonstrate a "mental fog" around emotional states (George & West, 2012). Defensive disconnection splits attachment distress from its source, maintaining organization but leaving the individual confused and uncertain (George & West, 2012). This pattern closely resembled Emma's responses to being alone in the real world; she quickly became unable to cope and directed anger toward others, suggesting confusion about the cause of her feelings.

Emma's response pattern to the dyadic stimuli was similar, as evidenced in her response to Bed[4]:

Lady in a bed. ... (What happened before?) *I don't know.* (What do you think the people are thinking or feeling?) *Shouting* (Shouting) (Can you tell me anymore?) No. (What happened next?) *I don't know.*	Disconnect Disconnect Disconnect

Note that Emma only identifies the adult in the picture, despite the clear depiction of a child character as well (the projected self). It is unusual in the AAP for individuals not to identify all the characters drawn in a scene. The failure to identify the projected self (the child) suggested that for Emma, separation and attachment-caregiving themes were bound up in intense anger (shouting) and that she experienced her needs as invisible to her caregivers. This may help explain her difficulty talking about her family; feeling "invisible" may have left her without a language to talk about their relationship. Her response may also explain the anger she directed toward her support workers. Being dependent on staff (like a dependent child) would likely have led her to experience them as attachment figures. As such, separations or threats to that care would unleash the anger we see in responses.

In Cemetery, the second to the last stimulus in the AAP set, the tension that Emma experienced with the increased activation of attachment almost "froze" her ability to respond. Of all her responses, this response was the closest to being constricted, except she was able to describe feelings:

(What is happening in this picture?) No. (What are they thinking or feeling?) *Angry* and sad. (Can you tell me more about that?) No. (What happened before?) No. (What happens next?) *I don't know*   —   Disconnect / Disconnect

This was the only story where Emma refused to provide elements for a story (i.e., saying "no" rather than her usual "I don't know"). This response shift suggested that Cemetery was more distressing for Emma than the other scenes. Even so, she was able to describe the character's feeling state as angry and sad, a pattern that was consistent with her other responses. Emma's response to Cemetery suggested that her reliance on cognitive disconnection was fragile at times. We could hypothesize that emotions connected to loss could tip her into a state of dysregulation at times of high stress or when she felt very alone.

Clinical application

Emma's AAP responses were sparse, but on deeper analysis, they did not appear to be purely an artifact of her ID. In other situations, she could speak in sentences and hold a basic conversation about various topics. However, when it came to talking about details related to her family, she exhibited similar difficulties as we saw on the AAP; when pressed, she deflected to "I don't know." This contrast suggested that in the face of difficult and painful affect, she became confused and passive, experiencing herself and her needs as invisible to caregivers. The paucity of information and the difficulties Emma seemed to have articulating memories or thoughts about her family illustrate how challenging it would have been to use interview-based assessment such as the Adult Attachment Interview (AAI, George et al., 1984) and emphasizes the value of the AAP in these circumstances.

Uncovering Emma's representation of self in relationships enabled us to reformulate Emma's relationships with support workers, who she likely experienced as attachment figures. Her jealousy and aggression were understood as reflecting her ambivalent state of mind, whereby she desired closeness but was confused about how to achieve this when she felt invisible. As a result, Emma pulled others in only to angrily push them away in the same pattern that Ainsworth described of anxious ambivalent infants (Ainsworth et al., 1978). The preoccupied-ambivalent pattern also suggested why Emma would flounder if left alone for too long; she needed the physical presence and scaffolding of caregivers to help regulate difficult feelings and prevent explosions. This attachment-based evaluation provided a view of Emma as needing more, not less, support and served as a counterpoint to previous attempts to reduce her support hours because of her behavior. Her repeated placement breakdowns could be conceived as reflecting an over-reliance on behavioral perspectives or blaming narratives (e.g., carers viewing her as manipulative) at the expense of considering the very real anxieties and fears of abandonment that she experienced when receiving care from others.

Feedback was given to Emma in person with the help of an easy-to-read letter covering key themes from her AAP in basic language. She appeared emotionally disconnected during this session, which could be due to her underlying defensive posture or her ID, but most likely an intersection of both. Emma's disconnecting defense of "not knowing" when faced with the self in relationships may be so ingrained that it will take time and patient interactions with caregivers to enable her to make connections between her experiences and her feelings.

Our main clinical intervention was via a training day for support workers to introduce the concepts of attachment and particularly how a preoccupied state of mind could result in a high need for reassurance, and a tendency for individuals to be combative and angry to draw people close. The formulation derived from Emma's AAP was used in conjunction with other assessments, including a functional analysis of her behavior, to update her Positive Behavior Support Plan. One essential guideline was for support workers to check in with Emma as soon as they started work to give Emma a sense that she was being thought about (i.e., not invisible) and provide a consistent message about who was available for her. We suggested that Emma be offered consistent times for guaranteed one on one support, to minimize her need to act out to draw others close. Emma's AAP showed that her representational self was full of sadness and anger, but that she was neither able to think about these feelings nor take constructive action when she was distressed. Support workers were therefore encouraged to validate and label feelings for Emma and link them to a source (e.g., "I wonder if you're feeling sad" or "it is annoying that you can't work with so-and-so today"). This process was thought to develop her ability to think and talk about these feelings in the contexts in which they appeared. Support workers were also guided in the use of accessible mood diaries, daily talk time, and ways of supporting Emma to develop constructive strategies to manage difficult feelings "in the moment" (e.g., soothing activities, mindfulness). When Emma was distressed, support workers were encouraged to maintain a calm and non-blaming stance. Should support workers need to leave for their safety, they were encouraged to return after a short interval and offer further support to reconnect and prevent Emma from feeling abandoned. The plan explicitly stated that support workers should avoid a critical tone or berating Emma after incidents to reduce further emotional entanglement and outrage.

The attachment approach introduced a new element to which support staff had not previously been exposed and moved away from locating the problem solely within Emma. It was not surprising, then, that initially, the team appeared defensive and angry at the training session, making it harder for them to see Emma's perspective. We found it essential to explicitly recognize how difficult and draining it must be to support Emma. The insights from the AAP coupled with a timeline of her life enabled staff to understand that Emma's behavior was not about them as people or their competency as carers. Using this attachment approach, they began to develop compassion for her. Later, the support organization commented that the training session had been a "turning point" for Emma's workers and that understanding her attachment needs had helped them to adjust their approach. As a result, they told us that Emma was now "in a much better place."

Grace

Grace, age 13, was referred to a community Child and Adolescent Mental Health Services team for children and young people with ID for help with high levels of emotional distress and behavioral challenges, the majority of which were directed toward her parents. Grace would shout at them and ask repetitive questions about past events, asking her parents to confirm multiple times when and where events happened. Bedtimes, which for children are separations from their attachment figures (Bowlby, 1973), also appeared fraught with Grace needing a high level of emotional support to settle into sleep. At times of high anxiety, Grace often sought assistance with eating and using the bathroom facilities, tasks that she was able to complete independently when she was less anxious. Her parents were exhausted by her constant demands and were struggling to cope.

The initial assessment consisted of interviews with Grace's parents and her school to get a developmental history and understand the background for Grace's presentation. Grace was observed at school, and we offered family sessions in the home to observe and assess family interaction patterns.

Background

Grace had several neurological and developmental conditions and lived in a challenging family context. She was diagnosed with Tuberous Sclerosis (TS), a rare genetic condition causing benign tumors to develop in different parts of the body, including the brain. TS is typically associated with various other conditions as well. Grace was also diagnosed with ID, epilepsy, and Autism Spectrum Disorder. She lived with her biological parents and her twin brother, with each family member also having complex health needs. Like Grace, her father had TS and epilepsy. Her twin brother had TS and mild ID. Grace's mother had a chronic pain condition that flared up unpredictably and could leave her incapacitated for up to a week at a time. As a result of her conditions, Grace attended a special educational unit within a mainstream secondary school in England.

Grace was an anxious child and tense separation experiences were prominent in her history. Grace had always shown high levels of anxiety on separation from her parents including when she started nursery school and when she initially commenced primary school. Since the age of 6, Grace was anxious about her mobility, choosing not to walk, or seeking supports and walking aids, despite no physical cause for these concerns. At the age of 8, allegations of parental abuse led to a sudden separation from her parents. Grace's aunt cared for her for two nights while the allegations were investigated by social services. The allegations were shown to be unfounded, and Grace returned to her family's care. Grace experienced a significant loss when she was 11 when her godmother died. Her godmother had been a key support to the family, and although her parents attended the funeral, Grace did not attend herself. Grace frequently referred to separation and loss in her daily conversation. For example, she continued to be upset about being separated from her parents at the time of the social services investigations and remained aggrieved that her parents had left her elsewhere to attend her godmother's funeral. Grace's distress about these events appeared fresh, with no sense of time or realization that these events had happened in the past.

The prominence of separation, loss, and anxiety in relationships with caregivers in the initial assessment pointed toward the importance of applying an attachment lens to understand Grace's clinical presentation. Her parents' disabilities combined with her brother's need for care also suggested that caregiver availability could be compromised. The AAP was offered to develop this initial psychological formulation beyond observable behavior and delve further into Grace's internal working model of attachment.

AAP assessment, classification, and analysis

Grace engaged well with the AAP. She was able to tell a story in response to each AAP scene, often mixed in with her rules of life or leakage into her own experience. Grace was classified as Unresolved. Her main organizing defense was deactivation with a particular focus on rules and social scripts.

Grace's "alone" stories allowed us to see the quality of Grace's relationships with others, which were impersonal and revealed her anger toward those in authority who attempted to exert power over her. This pattern was evidenced in Bench[5]:

She's putting her legs across because she's getting *angry*	Disconnect
and sad no not sad upset. She's at *PE* no she's not *PEing,*	Deactivate
she's at *swimming* and she's, that made out of plastic or?	
And she's um she had a *tantrum* because she won't let, she	Disconnect
won't do as hers told, she probably won't, she won't do	
as no *she won't do listen* to any *swimming* person	Deactivate
(What happened before?)	
don't know ...(what are the people thinking or feeling?)	Disconnect
said that girls sad and upset and she's *fed up* and she's um	Disconnect
she's she's upset and she's upset, *cross,* sad and *stressed*	Disconnect
and because *she won't do as her told.* The *lifeguard at*	Deactivate
swimming that's why she's in a right state, sometimes	
do I feel like that girl there or do I feel not like a normal	
person (What might happen next?) She'll probably, <u>go to</u>	Agency: action
<u>her room</u> and stay in her room until not stay in her room	
until teatime, and then when she after her tea <u>she goes</u>	Agency: action
<u>straight to bed</u> and think about her actions.	

Notice how Grace oscillates between the defensive disconnection (anger) and deactivation (adult authority via the lifeguard at swimming) as she tries to manage the situation. Eventually, the character acts by going to her room and "straight to bed," which contains the situation but also removes the possibility of her being connected with others. The "thinking" at the end of the story was a candidate for evaluation as the internalized secure base, but on closer analysis appeared to be connected only to actions, not to personal or relational topics. Grace's agency to change her situation appeared to be rooted in anger and defiance against authority.

The themes of authority and anger shifted in the direction of threat and pain as Grace's attachment system was increasingly activated by the alone AAP pictures. Neurological evidence suggests that Corner is the most stressful and distressing picture in the AAP battery (Buchheim et al., 2006). This was the case for Grace:

(What's going on in the picture?) A person, he's doing ...	
like <u>"don't hurt me"</u> or <u>"don't threaten"</u> or um............	Deactivate &
	Agency: action

> *don't know* (What happened before?) What you mean   Disconnect
> ***threatening me, what threatening on there?*** um I know   Trauma
> why the boy's ***threaten because the lady smacked the***   Trauma
> ***boy in the face kicked not kicked I mean smacked face***   Trauma
> ***pushed on the floor,*** ...and he and <u>*he say, "no no."*</u>   Deactivate &
> (What are the people thinking or feeling?) Sad, no, not   Agency: action
> sad, *cross, fed up, stressed, really angry.* (What might   Disconnect
> happen next?) I know why the boy's doing like that
> because he doesn't want his needles done because he was
> feeling like "please don't put needles, needles in my,"
> what's this called, yeh, "don't put needles in my arm,"
> that's why he's like that, he doesn't want his injections.

Grace's immediate response to Corner was a story of the projected self being terrorized by an adult. Both elements of her story, being smacked and the injection, involve potential pain. Threatened and angry, Grace's agency is activated, and she jumps into action by rejecting the threatening person (deactivation) to protect herself from potential harm. As in Bench, Grace's anger fuels deactivation and agency, thus enabling her to regain some sense of regulation. Although problematic in many ways, Grace's anger is also protective. Note too how Grace once again attempts to regulate by shifting her attention away from the story to explain the boy's actions via a social script (injections), allowing her to deactivate from the threat.

Grace's dyadic stories included themes of traumatic separation, death, and abuse. Again, she was able to remain regulated if she kept these events at a distance. For example, in Departure, which depicts potential separation fears, she shifted to a lengthy "personal logic" speech about how to say goodbye to someone who had died rather than complete the hypothetical story. Her Ambulance story concerned someone who died after being "smacked or collapsed," a trauma combined with a surreal state of being (i.e., derealization, see Chapter 4), but this was regulated by keeping the characters impersonal with no attachment relationship between them, and taking functional care of the dead body (i.e., an ambulance took the deceased to the graveyard).

Grace's distancing defenses and attentional maneuvering failed, however, when faced with the projected self and a mother figure in Bed. A family dynamic of punishment for misbehavior and potential abandonment plunged her into dysregulation, and this story was the source of her Unresolved classification[6]:

> The boy's going to bed because *her mum won't let her kiss*   Deactivate
> *goodnight or give her a cuddle because of his behavior,* he's
> upset because of his behavior, he's upset like a waaah upset
> and he, the person *the mum and the boy won't let cuddle the*   Deactivate
> *boy because of his attitude.* (What led up to the scene?)

He's *angry* and *fed up* and *stressed* and the boy *won't*	Disconnect
cuddle my mom because she's stressed the mum and she's *fed*	Deactivate
up. (Thinking or feeling?) *Angry, fed up, stressed, can't cope*	Disconnect
that means the boy *has to leave the house to live somewhere*	Trauma
else because mum and dad can't stick the boy,[5] if he can't	
get to sleep *he can't go out because of his behavior*. (Happens	Deactivate
next?) He, the boy is *won't get toys because of his behavior*.	
He won't get his toy cars because of his behavior and he	
won't go out because of his behaviors and he's *jumping up*	Deactivate
and down being moody.	Disconnect

This story showed what happened to Grace's defenses and her ability to regulate painful emotion when confronted with an attachment figure who deactivated their relationship by rejecting her need for comfort and emotional security. There was confusion between the character being a boy and "her," and at one moment during her storytelling she actually slipped into language speaking of her own mother (e.g. "my mum"). Her inability to manage the boundary between telling a story and her own life was evidence of how distressing rules, parental punishment, and perceived rejection were for her. Grace's awareness of her current family dynamic was evidenced throughout this story and suggested that on some level she knew that her parents were overwhelmed by her behavior; they were helpless and unable to cope. It is possible that this was linked to their serious health conditions, but regardless, Grace's stories suggested that she experienced them as abdicating their parental responsibilities as a direct result of her difficult behavior. Parental abdication is an attachment trauma (George & West, 2012). Grace's stories told us that this threat left her feeling alone, afraid, extremely angry, and dysregulated.

Clinical application

Grace's AAP responses spoke clearly to her experiences of the effects of separations and losses (sudden parental separation, her godmother's death). The AAP gave insights into her affect and behavior that had not been considered previously. Her angry defiance at authority was revealed as protective, keeping threatening affect at bay. The prominence of illness and fear (injections in Corner, traumatic death in Ambulance) was striking given her parents' health problems that at times rendered them incapacitated and unavailable. These experiences then elevated the meaning of separation in Grace's eyes. The rejection of a nighttime hug in Bed became the result of the character's difficult behavior. Even though not intrinsically dangerous, Grace experienced this as attachment trauma that she was not able to contain. Further, Grace's perspective-taking difficulty may have led her to feel personally responsible for her parents' struggles, as though her behavior, rather than their ill health, was the primary cause. Her threatened sense of self, evidenced in part by repeated requests for reassurance may have been Grace's attempts to keep her parents close and guard against loss. Her retreat to needing more physical care at times of distress may have been her way of guaranteeing that someone would be available to her. In sum, the AAP gave new meaning to Grace's presentation that went beyond listing a set of behavioral challenges and toward understanding her behavior as an expression of overwhelming anger and fear.

Communicating these new insights to Grace's family required great sensitivity. The implication that Grace's presentation was linked to parental helplessness and abdication had the potential to be extremely painful for the family. Careful consideration was given to the content and format of the feedback to make this clinically helpful for the family and to avoid prompting feelings of blame or criticism. The impact of Grace's social communication difficulties was crucial here, in terms of considering how this may have effected the development of reciprocal interactions with her parents, and perhaps led her to develop misattributions about her parents' health.

We discussed Grace's AAP with her and her family in two stages. COVID pandemic restrictions in place at the time necessitated that this discussion took place online, which unfortunately complicated matters as Grace struggled to engage with online sessions. We constructed an easy-to-read letter for Grace, which included pictures to support her understanding. We held a second session with Grace's parents, which was supported with another letter and included pictures and diagrams. The AAP helped reframe some of Grace's parents' concerns. They said that they found it difficult to establish a clear reciprocal connection with her when she was repetitive, shouting, or throwing things. They felt as though they could not "tune in" to her. We explained this behavior as an expression of her underlying separation worries and fears, making explicit links to Grace's prior separation experiences. There was further discussion about the extent to which themes of loss and illness dominated Grace's underlying anxiety, leaving her frequently overwhelmed and dysregulated. The possibility that she may fear losing her parents through illness allowed a deeper exploration of her underlying anxiety.

Grace's parents engaged well with this feedback and reported feeling understood and validated. They felt that the AAP had highlighted patterns of interacting that they found challenging to manage and that this enabled them to better understand the fears beneath Grace's observable behavior. By focusing on what Grace brought to their interactions and the intersection with her developmental disabilities, her parents were able to engage in this discussion without feeling blamed or judged for their parenting. This discussion lessened their defensiveness and made them more open to discourse with clinicians. The AAP made it possible for them to explore the extent to which Grace focused on rules and behavior, with the implication that she often experienced authority without emotional connection. The family was facilitated to think about ways of establishing a more meaningful emotional connection with Grace, and both acknowledging and reassuring her concerns about separation, loss, and illness. Greater emotional containment could enable Grace to build on the potential seen in her AAP. Her character in Bench had been depicted as thinking but without genuine emotional connection. Clinicians hypothesized that if Grace experienced greater emotional containment from those caring for her, she may well be able to develop this potential and integrate thoughtful activity with emotional experiences.

Grace's case describes the first known use of the AAP with an adolescent with ID. Previously, the AAP has only been used with those with ID aged 18 and over. This suggests that there may be wider scope to use the AAP to support the assessment of internal working models in children and young people within this cohort. The AAP allows for a more direct assessment of attachment-related thoughts and feelings than is possible through other means of attachment assessment which are more reliant on a higher level of verbal ability and use of verbal prompts (e.g., Child Attachment Interview; Target et al., 2003). We propose that further research on using the use of the AAP in young people with ID would be fruitful.

Conclusion

Both of the cases presented in this chapter suggested an interplay between ID and attachment experiences, illustrating how confusion (Emma) and social communication difficulties (Grace) complicated experiences of separation, loss, and illness. These hypotheses suggest that ID and attachment influence each other, creating a "both-and" rather than an "either-or" situation. This bears similarities to the hypotheses of Rutgers et al. (2004) and Schuengel and Janssen (2006) (see above).

It is common for people with ID to be experienced as behaviorally challenging by their caregivers, but scant attention has been given to how such interactions can impact the person's sense of themselves as worthy of care. Use of the AAP meant that clinical formulations were based on internal working models, rather than observable or reported behavior alone. This enabled the formulations to focus more precisely on the elements of attachment state of mind that underpinned distress. Greater precision in formulation enables intervention to be more focused and to connect more meaningfully to those affected by the distress. Using the AAP allowed others to "step inside" the internal world of the person with ID, and appreciate thoughts, feelings, and fears that may be too difficult to acknowledge or articulate. For a population that has usually been judged by observable behavior alone, this represents a welcome advance.

Notes

1 "Safeguarding" is the UK term for the process designed to protect children and vulnerable adults from abuse and neglect.
2 "Key-words" carry information and are the words one needs to understand in order to convey the exact meaning of a sentence.
3 Italics = defenses
4 Italics = defenses
5 Italics = defenses; underline = capacity to act
6 Italics = defenses; bold = trauma

References

Bateman, L. (2020). *Exploring attachment in adults with intellectual disability* [Unpublished doctoral dissertation]. University of Liverpool, UK.

Bowlby, J. (1980). *Attachment and loss: Vol. 3: Loss: Sadness and depression.* Basic Books.

Buchheim, A., Erk, S., George, C., Kaechele, H., Ruchsow, M., Spitzer, M., Kircher, T., Walter, H. (2006). Measuring attachment representation in an fMRI environment: A pilot study. *Psychopathology, 39*(3), 144–152. https://doi.org/10.1159/000091800

Fletcher, H. K., Flood, A., & Hare, D. (Eds.) (2016). *Attachment in intellectual and developmental disability: A clinician's guide to practice and research.* Wiley.

Gallichan, D. J., & George, C. (2014). Assessing attachment status in adults with intellectual disabilities: The potential of the adult attachment projective picture system. *Advances in Mental Health and Intellectual Disabilities, 8*(2), 103–119. https://doi.org/10.1108/amhid-10-2012-0004

Gallichan, D.J, & George, C. (2016). Attachment trauma and pathological mourning in adults with intellectual disabilities. In H. K. Fletcher, A. Flood, & D. J. Hare (Eds.), *Attachment in intellectual and developmental disability: A clinician's guide to practice and research* (pp. 197–222). Wiley.

Gallichan, D. J., & George, C. (2018). The Adult Attachment Projective Picture System: a pilot study of inter-rater reliability and face validity with adults with intellectual disabilities. *Advances in Mental Health and Intellectual Disabilities, 12*(2), 57–66. https://doi.org/10.1108/amhid-11-2017-0036

George, C., Kaplan, N., & Main, M. (1984/1985/1996). The adult attachment interview [Unpublished manuscript]. University of California, Berkeley.

Horner-Johnson, W., & Drum, C. E. (2006). Prevalences of maltreatment of people with intellectual disabilities: A review of recently published research. *Mental Retardation and Developmental Disabilities Research Reviews, 12* (1), 57–69. https://doi.org/10.10002/mrdd.20097.

Lyons-Ruth, K., & Jacobwitz, D. (2016). Attachment disorganization from infancy to adulthood: neurobiological correlates, parenting contexts, and pathways to disorder. In J. Cassidy & P. Shaver (Eds.), *Handbook of attachment: Theory, research, and clinical applications* (3rd ed., pp. 667–695). Guildford Press.

Rutgers, A. H., Bakermans- Kranenburg, M. J., van IJzendoorn, M. H., & Van Berckleaer-Onnes, I. A. (2004). Autism and attachment: a meta-analytic review. *Journal of Child Psychology and Psychiatry, 45*(6), 1123–1134. https://doi.org/10.1111/j.1469-7610.2004.t01-1-00305.x

Schuengel, C., & Janssen, C. (2006). People with mental retardation and psychopathology: Stress, affect regulation and attachment. A review. *International Review of Research in Mental Retardation, 32,* 229–260. https://doi.org/10.1016/S0074-7750(06)32008-3

Sinason, V. (1992). *Mental handicap and the human condition: New approaches from the Tavistock.* Free Association Books.

Target, M., Fonagy, P., Shmueli-Goetz, Y. (2003). Attachment representations in school-age children: The development of the child attachment interview (CAI). *Journal of Child Psychotherapy, 29*(2) 171–186. https://doi.org/10.1080/0075417031000138433.

World Health Organization Europe. (n.d.). Definition: intellectual disability   https://www.euro.who.int/en/health-topics/noncommunicable-diseases/mental-health/news/news/2010/15/childrens-right-to-family-life/definition-intellectual-disability

Part 4
Adolescents and parents

12 Does therapy matter for adolescents in the foster care system?

Linda Webster, David Joubert, and Ashley Petersen

Many children and adolescents in the foster care system have experienced what is known as complex or developmental trauma, trauma that is the result of interpersonal violence and exploitation, including neglect and abuse (D'Andrea et al., 2012; Pearlman & Curtois, 2005). van der Kolk (2005) argues that the interpersonal trauma in child maltreatment during critical developmental periods has a far-reaching negative impact on cognitive, social-emotional, and interpersonal domains. D'Andrea et al. (2012) refer to the range of maltreatment experiences considered interpersonal violence, including physical, sexual, and emotional abuse.

Because of the interpersonal nature of the violence of child maltreatment, attachment theory is a powerful construct for understanding the impact of the trauma and conceptualizing interventions. From an attachment perspective, attachment figures who induce fear and betrayal, child maltreatment is conceived as failed protection (George & Solomon, 2008). The Adult Attachment Projective Picture System (AAP) is an empirically supported and theory-informed assessment that provides understanding about specific aspects of an individual's state of mind regarding attachment. Thus, it offers clinicians a unique tool to help inform interventions that address many aspects of the attachment system, including defensive processes. It also seems uniquely poised for measuring essential components of complex trauma associated with disruptions or adversity in the attachment relationship. The following case discusses how information from the AAP can be directly translated into interventions in the therapeutic context for an adolescent who had experienced sexual abuse, abandonment, betrayal, loss of her siblings, and rejection by caregivers, all sequelae of complex trauma.

Maddie: A case study

Maddie was the first of three children born to her parents and had a younger sister and a younger brother and an older half-brother, and two younger half-sisters, all born to the same mother. There was a history of disruption in housing and caretaking. For example, Maddie experienced severe neglect as a younger child and was left in hotel rooms to care for

DOI: 10.4324/9781003215431-16

her siblings. Her father sexually abused her from the age of six to nine, and later the family (her paternal aunt and uncle) asked her to lie about the abuse so that her father wouldn't go to jail. As a result, her mother's failed protection and abdication were compounded by another betrayal (being asked to lie) associated with numerous adverse outcomes in the complex trauma literature (e.g., D'Andrea et al., 2012).

At approximately age ten, she and her two full siblings were placed in the care of their maternal aunt. Unfortunately, the aunt put her own needs before those of the children, and the children were expected to and were reinforced for care for the aunt's emotional needs. Maddie lived with them for five years before they eventually requested that she be moved due to her acting-out behavior. Following her departure from the home, her aunt and uncle did not allow her to contact her siblings and essentially cut off all communication. She was placed into a foster home, but she did not last there long due to drinking alcohol, taking drugs, and staying out late. She was also suspended multiple times from school for fighting and was failing all but two of her classes. She moved into the home of a girlfriend from school, which contained the mother of her friend, her friend, and her friend's two younger siblings.

When she began therapy with the third author, she admitted to having anger problems and stated that she was angry "70% of the time." She denied symptoms of depression, mania, and Post-Traumatic Stress Disorder. She admitted to having been suicidal while living with her aunt and uncle, but not currently. She abused drugs and alcohol and engaged in unprotected sex with multiple partners and seemed disconnected when speaking to her therapist about her experience. All of these are indications of complex trauma. Shortly after she began therapy, the therapist and social worker requested a psychological evaluation for diagnostic clarification to inform therapeutic and possible medication intervention. The therapist wanted to ensure that an attachment assessment was a component of the evaluation given Maddie's history of abandonment and abuse and rejection by primary caregivers.

Adult Attachment Projective Picture System

Maddie's attachment classification on the AAP was Unresolved. Main and Goldwyn (1984) define an unresolved state of mind regarding attachment as a form of psychological disorganization involving multiple (segregated) systems of attachment kept outside of conscious awareness. Segregation is a form of extreme defensive process in response to severe perceived threats to the self and protective failure, including loss and abuse (Bowlby, 1980; George & West, 2012). The traumatic experience, including any associated feelings of fear, helplessness, abandonment, and isolation, is segregated, or separated off from conscious awareness as a protective mechanism against a state of dysregulation. The link between attachment disorganization and maltreatment is well documented (e.g., Cyr et al., 2010). Here is Maddie's unresolved response to the Child in the Corner picture stimulus[1].

He looks like he's in … what do those people do the box thingies… like the entertainers that do like the …I don't know what they're called…*or like it looks like he's trying to mess around or he's trying to get out of something,* but it doesn't look like a box even, so I don't know. There's like barely anything on this page, there's like a person, looking down on the ground behind him, and his hands are up.	Disconnect
This one's weird. He's looking at *something on the group or like on the wall,* but there's nothing even there except for this, and I don't even think that's a part of the picture. I really don't know about the feelings on these ones because it doesn't show the faces or their emotion… so it's hard for me to just pop one up in the head on and just like put it on the picture, 'cause I don't have a wild imagination like that. He'll carry on with his day, he's doing something for just	Disconnected trauma
five second and then he's just *going to move on.*	Disconnect

Consistent with individuals who have experienced abuse and maltreatment, Maddie's response to the stimulus depicts her struggle to make sense of the story and contain the painful and overwhelming emotion that is evoked. Her narrative is limited to describing the character and dwells on her distress. In this context, she appears to be particularly sensitive to the absence of details she could use to anchor herself in reality.

Ultimately, Maddie remains unable to regulate the emotional distress caused by the activation of her attachment system. Instead of being able to engage in constructive action to regain her equilibrium (i.e., grounding), the projected self is described as resorting to impulsive behavior in an attempt to move past or gloss over the emotional distress. She never addresses how the character might change or resolve the situation. There is no indication of how Maddie might manage her feelings of isolation and emptiness. Maddie has a long history of using impulsive acting-out and self-destructive behaviors as her primary method of managing her emotional distress and feelings of isolation; however, they are only temporarily effective and cannot resolve the underlying abuse, abandonment, and failed protection that haunts her. Tragically, her impulsive attempts to avoid the feelings of isolation she experienced by engaging in sex with multiple partners contributed to her trauma reaction (disconnection of the experience) and her sense of isolation.

Of importance for therapy is a closer look at the other unique components of the AAP coding system. These provide a more contextualized view of defenses and strengths that may be utilized in the therapeutic process. The following sections step the reader through a discussion of the strengths and problems revealed in Maddie's attachment representation concerning the conceptual categories used to code the AAP (see Chapter 1).

Agency

Maddie's responses to the four alone pictures coded for agency demonstrated the full range of agency, including no agency, capacity to act, and one instance of an internalized secure base. The following is her response to Cemetery[2]:

Looks like one of his *friends or family* died. He's at a	Disconnect
cemetery... somebody died ... *it could have been an*	Disconnect
*accident, or somebody could have **killed themselves***	Trauma
or something happened, or that person passed away.	
He looks like he's ***visiting*** ... and that person has	Trauma
been dead for a long time, and he loo-. Well, he	
doesn't really have any emotion on his face is what	
I am saying, but like, what his body language is, is	
he's *thinking about that person,* he's sad that they're	Agency: internalized
gone but he's *past the point of crying because they've*	secure base
been gone for a long time, and he's just like *thinking*	Deactivate
about that person and the memories that they've had,	Agency: internalized
like by his body language. He'll like put roses, no, he	secure base
doesn't have roses in his hand. He'll <u>go home,</u> or like,	Agency: action
I don't know, <u>he'll just go home.</u>	

Early in her response, she states, *somebody could have killed themselves,* a segregated systems marker. Her narrative demonstrates the importance of this relationship in the internalized secure base when she references the character as thinking about the individual who passed away. The internalized secure base involves a type of mental activity. The person draws upon her internal resources to explore her inner world and experience (George & West, 2011, see Chapter 1). It bears a close relationship to concepts such as reflective self function (Fonagy et al., 1991) and mentalization (Fonagy et al., 2018). These concepts have shown reliable associations with psychotherapy outcomes (Fonagy & Bateman, 2006), affect regulation (Mohaupt et al., 2006), empathy (Choi-Kain & Gunderson, 2008), and cognitive and adaptive flexibility (Lopez & Brennan, 2000). The internalized secure base in the Cemetery story helps Maddie regain emotional homeostasis and points to her capacity to value and emotionally invest in relationships, all of which are considered positive aspects of Maddie's functioning.

Although the integration evidenced in Maddie's response to Cemetery is encouraging, the overall pattern of agency of self in Maddie's protocol suggests that internal or external conflicts associated with attachment are likely to be managed through action rather than thoughtful exploration. And as seen in her Corner story, intense activation of the attachment system risks hindering her ability to access her internalized secure base or take constructive action to contain emotional distress. Instead, she resorts to impulsive, poorly planned, or regressive behaviors to cope. This move from capacity to act to acting out is exemplified in her Corner story (see above) and her sexualized behavior and substance abuse.

Connectedness

Despite the importance Maddie places on relationships, her early interactions with caregivers have impacted her ability to trust others and feel connected to them in a meaningful way. In her response to the Window stimulus, there is no mention of connecting to others. Attachment figures limit her autonomy and prevent her from engaging with the outside world. In Bench, she references a fight but does not repair the relationship. Interestingly, the only people mentioned are attachment figures with no reference to peers, which is arguably vital at her age and reflects her difficulty with friendships. In both cases, the interactions are limited to functional relationships, lacking authentic, meaningful connections.

The absence of connectedness in a protocol is significant in several ways. First, it points to maladaptive schema regarding attachment relationships and minimal expectations from significant others. Second, Maddie's AAP protocol suggests that she views attachment figures limiting her autonomy. Third, a capacity to connect in a meaningful way is an important asset directly relevant to psychotherapy, both as a target and as an outcome. Maddie had not experienced others as trustworthy and capable of sensitive responding, so building trust in the therapeutic relationship was critical to helping her resolve her trauma and improve adaptive functioning. The therapist needed to connect with Maddie on a deeper level. They needed to see her, understand her, and help her see herself for who she truly is, not for what others have shown her or told her so far in her life.

Synchrony

Consistent with connectedness, Maddie's responses on the three dyadic picture stimuli only showed functional synchrony. There is no mutual reciprocal interaction between the characters or any evidence of sensitive caregiving by an attachment figure. In Departure, unspecified adults (i.e., not an adult attachment dyad) are traveling together. Like other stories in the protocol, the emphasis appears to be on leaving rather than engaging in reciprocal activity. The following is her response to Ambulance, which illustrates her difficulty viewing attachment figures as sensitive and responsive[3]:

This looks like a *nurse* ... and this looks like a kid. I don't	Deactivate
know what they are doing. That looks like an ambulance	Disconnect
that like took one of his family members in it or something	*Settles on nurse*
like that, or like *I don't know*, or like, something could	Disconnect
be happening to the neighbor, and then him and his mom	
are watching outside, but that looks like a *nurse* so they	Deactivate
could be in a hospital. *Somebody could have got hurt or*	
somebody's getting hurt or going to get hurt or... yeah. She	Disconnect
looks like she's trying to like comfort him and he's kinda	
just like *relaxed* and stuff... like the kid looks sad and that	Disconnect
guy looks like he's just trying to get his *job* done. They'll	Deactivate
carry on with their day. *Do what they normally would do.*	Deactivate

It is interesting that Maddie first identifies the adult character in this story as a nurse, then changes her mind and identifies the character as the *mom*. Despite her efforts to make this an attachment story, she cannot hold onto the image or idea of the mom being present for her child (i.e., the projected self) in a time of potential distress. She lands on it being a nurse who comforts the kid, which is considered deactivated functional care by a professional playing a role according to a social script.

Maddie's response to the Bed picture does include a mother figure; however, she is engaged in restraining or constraining the child (i.e., projected self.) The mother's behavior is misattuned, intrusive, and disruptive of the child's emotional state to the extent that the child has to ask for help. This caregiver-child interaction is consistent with Maddie's experience of caregivers as dysregulating rather than helping regulate affect.

Overall, Maddie's responses indicate that her caregiving experiences did not include mutual enjoyment, reciprocity, or consistent or reliable sensitive care. We can see from Maddie's dyadic stories that she has not learned how to negotiate her needs with the needs of others in close relationships because she had no real experience of this in her childhood and adolescence. This pattern highlights the importance of a positive therapeutic relationship with her therapist and regular and ongoing work with the caregiver to help her understand the nature of Maddie's traumatic, resistant response to her caregiving.

Defensive processes

The therapist's evaluation of the defensive processes pattern that emerges on the AAP can help determine their approach to working with a client. As shown in the story examples, Maddie's main defensive strategy is cognitive disconnection, which typically appears as mental fog created by frequent *I don't know* statements and the portrayal of multiple possibilities to account for story events. The effect of the disconnection is also evidenced in Maddie's struggle to name events and individuals in her responses. This pattern has been shown in other cases of children and youth in the foster care system (Jankowska et al., 2015; Webster & Hackett, 2011) and is not surprising given the amount of uncertainty in these children's lives, particularly regarding the instability of access to attachment figures. Maddie's pattern also evidenced disconnected anger in the Bench story, depicted as fighting with others. Maddie's confused disconnected fog serves to obscure conscious connections between her anger and deficiencies in attachment figure care.

Maddie attempts to distance herself from attachment distress through the use of deactivation. As seen in the Ambulance story, deactivation is an effective defense for her at times. Still, as attachment distress increases, she cannot maintain this strategy and falls back into using cognitive disconnection and confusion, as seen in her Bed story. This failure has implications for therapy, as a goal would be to help her maintain emotional distance when she becomes emotionally overwhelmed.

Finally, the segregated systems present in her responses indicate attachment trauma dysregulation (see Chapter 4). Her attempt to disconnect from her feelings of personal loss in Cemetery fails, and she is flooded by such intensity that she suggests the person may have died by suicide. Maddie can regain her footing and regulate herself by taking constructive action in this story. However, she cannot recover from the emergence of traumatic material in response to Corner, where she describes feelings of emptiness and isolation that echo the abuse and abandonment that she experienced. The Corner stimulus overwhelms her regulating defenses (disconnection and deactivation) and leaves her in a place of fear, isolation, and dysregulation. This failure to anchor herself – regain emotional homeostasis – leads to her Unresolved classification.

Of importance to discuss is Maddie's response to a discussion of the results of the AAP. After the testing, Maddie's therapist discussed the AAP results with her. Maddie was resistant to the discussion and feedback. Throughout this discussion, she rolled her eyes, interrupted the therapist with tangential statements or questions, and failed to engage. When asked about the stories and her experience, Maddie reported that the pictures were "weird and boring." If we were coding an AAP, "boring" would be considered a form of defensive disconnection. Thus, it seems noteworthy that Maddie's response to the therapist concerning her experience was consistent with the overarching regulating defense we observed in her stories.

AAP-based therapy goals and outcomes

Based on the information gleaned from Maddie's AAP and her history of disrupted attachment relationships and trauma, it became clear that the primary focus of therapy should be on building a trusting relationship between Maddie and her therapist. Without a safe holding environment, no other work could be done. Bowlby (1988) emphasized the therapist's role as acting as a secure base, providing a safe place with the therapist as a model of a surrogate attachment figure for the client to explore experience and affect.

The AAP also honed in on several other areas to target Maddie's therapy. One was to improve Maddie's agency by helping her develop the skills she needed to take positive, constructive actions in her life instead of turning to more self-destructive behaviors. As we saw in Maddie's AAP, her ability to regulate her emotions when distressed was compromised, thus obstructing her from taking constructive action or from being able to think things through. This dynamic could also be seen in her life and was often reenacted in the therapy room. At the beginning of many sessions, Maddie's affect appeared dysregulated, which seemed to disrupt her thought process and her ability to collaborate with her therapist when trying to come up with an action plan. Maddie needed to develop some emotional regulation strategies to increase her capacity for thoughtful action.

One approach that Maddie's therapist took to help her manage her feelings was to bolster her deactivating defenses. Together, they worked on developing problem-solving strategies using different forms of communication (i.e., writing letters) to help Maddie adaptively express her emotions. Additionally, Maddie was encouraged to think about her relationships and separate or distance herself from distressing ones. This intervention was helpful because it gave Maddie time to preempt meltdowns and consider behavior she would like to use to approach a future relationship or conflict. They also worked on stress reduction techniques. Stress increased Maddie's frustration and intense reactions to situations and people and usurped the agency needed to manage day-to-day stress, for example, school performance and home life. Medication was also helpful in lending executive control so that Maddie was more effective in inhibiting knee-jerk trauma reactions to stressors.

Another goal was to improve Maddie's capacity for relatedness – connectedness and synchrony – to combat feelings of isolation and disruptive anger, especially with her foster mother and sister (the caregiver's biological child). The therapist arranged several meetings between Maddie and her foster mother and her foster sister occasionally. The goal here was fostering perspective-taking by helping each understand safety and protection as viewed by the other. Mutual perspective-taking was needed if these relationships were to become balanced (i.e., a goal-corrected partnership, Bowlby, 1982). For example, there needed to be a balance between autonomy and independence regarding protection to promote adaptive development while also containing Maddie's propensity for destructive acting-out behavior.

The foster mother, a first-time foster mother, had unrealistic expectations for their relationship and Maddie's behavior. Additionally, she was unprepared for Maddie's assault on her caregiving. For example, when Maddie first moved in, the foster mother told the therapist that she "loves" Maddie and planned to be strict with her since she knew that "she can lie and do bad things." Shortly afterward, Maddie was in trouble for lying and sneaking out of the house. Bowlby (1982) placed great emphasis on the effects of actual experience on attachment behavior. From this perspective, Maddie's behaviors were extreme attachment signals of desperation and distress (Allen, 2008) when she learned that her siblings had been adopted by her aunt and uncle and that her failing grades required her to repeat a year of high school. As with most caregivers who do not know about attachment, the foster mother focused on managing the acting-out behavior and not its source. The therapist helped them negotiate realistic expectations and improve communication through active listening and role play.

Following three months of intensive relationship work, the foster mother and social worker saw that Maddie's behavior and grades at school improved, and she argued less. However, a few weeks later, Maddie complained that her foster mother was "taking things out on her," and problems of sibling jealousy reemerged. The therapist continued to offer family sessions with Maddie, her foster sister, and her mother. The sessions helped, but relationship dysregulation continued, as would be predicted by her unresolved state of mind regarding attachment.

Another therapeutic goal was addressing Maddie's reliance on the defensive exclusion processes associated with cognitive disconnection. Addressing this goal involved helping her make connections between affect and its source and to engage the prefrontal cortex in the inhibition of impulsive behavior. The therapist eventually wanted to begin some trauma work, but Maddie needed stabilization first because she was still very easily upset by her aunt.

Maddie developed a strong therapeutic bond with her therapist, so another therapeutic goal was to help her understand how to use relationships for affect regulation. In addition to her childhood experiences of sexual abuse, abandonment, and rejection, she experienced another trauma while in therapy. Maddie's father was released from jail and, while she did not have contact with him, this was frightening for her, and this fear entered the therapeutic relationship. His anticipated presence frightened her. Maddie put immense trust in the therapist during this vulnerable and scary time. Holidays, especially Christmas, dysregulated her as well. She missed her siblings, plus Maddie was her siblings' primary caregiver. Her aunt continually interfered with her relationships with them. The therapist encouraged Maddie to write her feelings and thoughts in letters to her siblings as a controlled affect regulation strategy. Maddie's child welfare worker made sure Maddie's siblings got the letters, and she was pleased to receive their return letters.

Approximately a year into therapy, Maddie completed another AAP to determine progress in her representation of attachment and relationships. Her classification had shifted to Preoccupied. Although better regulated, this AAP showed that cognitive disconnection continued to be Maddie's primary regulating defense, and she still struggled with a mental fog about the meaning of attachment events. However, the new AAP did show that Maddie had responded positively to her attachment-based therapeutic intervention. She had developed a view of herself as being able to take positive action (capacity to act) and some increased ability to think through attachment dilemmas (internalized secure base). Her stories portrayed more connectedness, reciprocity, and caregiver sensitivity and attunement.

Another therapeutic goal had been to confront her reliance on disconnecting defenses to help Maddie make clear conscious connections between her feelings and their source. The AAP demonstrated some progress toward this goal; however, the appearance of her biological mother shortly after testing highlighted the fragility of cognitive disconnection as a regulating defense. Maddie struggled to establish a relationship with her mother. Still, she was derailed when confronted with the presence of the mother, who had failed to protect her from her father's abuse and memories of role-reversed parentification. Her already fragile relationship with her foster mother began to deteriorate beyond repair. Maddie reacted by feeling that she was being treated unfairly. Her foster mother said openly that she "didn't want [Maddie] in the house if the undesirable behavior continued." Her misbehavior resulted in coercive threats of abandonment to ensure compliance. From an attachment perspective, Maddie's actions were attempts to escape her intensely painful feelings of her mother's rejection and abandonment. Again threatened with abandonment, these feelings now generalized to her foster mother.

Ending the therapeutic relationship

Despite the efforts to salvage the relationship between Maddie and her foster mother, Maddie left after 18 months to live with a friend following an argument with her foster sister. During that time, she began throwing objects in the house. There was a mutual understanding from both Maddie and her foster mother, supported by the therapist that the foster home was not the best fit for Maddie's needs. The foster mother acknowledged that she had unrealistic expectations of her ability to provide for Maddie's emotional needs. Maddie was able to express her desire to leave the home, as well as the anger she felt toward her foster mother. She had difficulty, however, acknowledging any other feelings besides anger. A month later, Maddie told her therapist that she had texted her foster mother, telling her that she still loved her even though they had fought before she left. She was disappointed that her foster mother did not respond, which constituted another attachment trauma and produced feelings of abandonment. The following month Maddie came to therapy after missing two sessions, reporting that she had moved to another city approximately 45 minutes away; attending therapy required a complex route using public transportation. Despite her traumatic history of abuse, rejection, and abandonment, it is quite remarkable that Maddie took a train and a bus to meet the therapist with whom she had established a positive working alliance and trusting relationship. Although Maddie wanted to continue with her therapist, it became clear that the distance and transportation were insurmountable challenges. She lived in transitional housing with three roommates and thought she might be pregnant. The therapist recommended to the child welfare worker and stressed to Maddie that she find a new therapist closer to where she lived. Maddie and her biological mother reconnected in their last session, but other outcomes are not known.

Conclusion

This chapter illustrates the use of a fine-grained analysis of the unique features of the AAP coding and classification system for therapeutic intervention and as a potential means to measure the effectiveness of therapeutic intervention using a very challenging case of complex trauma. The AAP gives the clinician access to assess key attachment components that map onto the challenges evident in complex trauma, including defensive processing. A client's particular defensive processing pattern, along with the qualitative and idiosyncratic personal information in the story responses, illuminates a client's state of mind. For Maddie, this information allowed for interventions that could target specific behaviors and defenses in the context of attachment and other filial relationships. The measurement of agency as an internalized secure base is a unique aspect of the AAP. While central to the therapeutic goals of most therapies, it is arguably critical to the treatment of complex trauma (e.g., Luyten et al., 2020). Maddie's case also highlights the importance of developing a trusting, secure base therapeutic relationship as the primary mechanism to help a client improve emotion regulation and prevent being triggered and becoming dysregulated. This case illustrates the fragility of the Preoccupied state of mind and how easily the defense can fail in the advent of additional attachment trauma. Maddie's setback when confronted with her biological mother demonstrates that the development of and change in attachment trauma is a long-term process and not something that is easily or quickly addressed (e.g., Ruff et al., 2019).

Notes

  1 Italics = defenses; bold = trauma
  2 Italics = defenses; bold = trauma
  3 Italics = defenses

References

Allen, J. P. (2008). *The attachment system in adolescence.* Guilford Press.

Ayoub, C. C., O'Connor, E., Rappolt-Schlichtmann, G., Fischer, K. W., Rogosch, F. A., Toth, S. L., & Cicchetti, D. (2006). Cognitive and emotional differences in young maltreated children: A translational application of dynamic skill theory. *Development and Psychopathology, 18*(3), 679–706. https://doi.org/10.1017/S0954579406060342

Bowlby, J. (1980). *Attachment and loss: Vol. 3. Loss.* Basic Books. [Original publication, 1969]

Bowlby, J. (1982). *Attachment and loss: Vol. 1. Attachment.* Basic Books.

Bowlby, J. (1988). *A secure base.* Basic Books.

Choi-Kain, L. W., & Gunderson, J. G. (2008). Mentalization: Ontogeny, assessment, and application in the treatment of borderline personality disorder. *American Journal of Psychiatry, 165*(9), 1127–1135. https://doi.org/10.1176/appi.ajp.2008.07081360

Cyr, C., Euser, E. M., Bakermans-Kranenburg, M. J., & van IJzendoorn, M. H. (2010). Attachment security and disorganization in maltreating and high-risk families: A series of meta-analyses. *Development and Psychopathology, 22*(1), 87–108. https://doi.org/10.1017/S0954579409990289

D'Andrea, W., Ford, J., Stolbach, B., Spinazzola, J., & van der Kolk, B. (2012). Understanding interpersonal trauma in children: Why we need a developmentally appropriate trauma diagnosis. *American Journal of Orthopsychiatry, 82*(2), 187–200. https://doi.org/10.1111/j.1939-0025.2012.01154.x

Fonagy, P., Gergely, G., & Jurist, E. L. (Eds.). (2018). *Affect regulation, mentalization and the development of the self.* Routledge.

Fonagy, P., Steele, M., Steele, H., Moran, G. S., & Higgitt, A. C. (1991). The capacity for understanding mental states: The reflective self in parent and child and its significance for security of attachment. *Infant Mental Health Journal, 12*(3), 201–218. https://doi.org/10.1002/1097-0355(199123)12:3<201::AID-IMHJ2280120307>3.0.CO;2-7

George, C., & Solomon, J. (2008). The caregiving system: A behavioral systems approach to parenting. In J. Cassidy & P. R. Shaver (Eds.), *Handbook of attachment: Theory, research, and clinical applications* (2nd ed., pp. 833–856). Guilford Press.

George, C., & West, M. (2011). The adult attachment projective picture system: integrating attachment into clinical assessment. *Journal of Personality Assessment, 93*(5), 407–416. https://doi.org/10.1080/00223891.2011.594133

George, C., & West, M. (2012). *The adult attachment projective picture system.* Guilford Press.

Jankowska, A. M., Lewandowska-Walter, A., Chalupa, A. A., Jonak, J., Duszynski, R., & Mazurkiewicz, N. (2015). Understanding the relationships between attachment styles, locus of control, school maladaptation, and depression symptoms among students in foster care. In *School Psychology Forum, 9*(1), 44–58.

Lawrence, V. A., & Lee, D. (2014). An exploration of peoples' experiences of compassion-focused therapy for trauma, using interpretive phenomenological analysis. *Clinical Psychology and Psychotherapy, 21*(6), 495–507. https://doi.org/10.1002/cpp.1854

Lopez, F. G., & Brennan, K. A. (2000). Dynamic processes underlying adult attachment organization:Toward an attachment theoretical perspective on the healthy and effective self. *Journal of Counseling Psychology, 47*(3), 283–300. https://doi.org/10.1037//0022-0167.47.3.283

Luyten, P., Campbell, C., & Fonagy, P. (2020). Borderline personality disorder, complex trauma, and problems with self and identity: A social-communicative approach. *Journal of Personality, 88*(1), 88–105. https://doi.org/10.1111/jopy.12483

Main, M., & Goldwyn, R. (1984). Predicting rejection of her infant from mother's representation of her own experience: Implications for the abused-abusing intergenerational cycle. *Child Abuse and Neglect, 8*(2), 203–217. https://doi.org/10.1016/0145-2134(84)90009-7

Mohaupt, H., Holgersen, H., Binder, P. E., & Nielsen, G. H. (2006). Affect consciousness or mentalization? A comparison of two concepts with regard to affect development and affect regulation. *Scandinavian Journal of Psychology, 47*(4), 237–244. https://doi.org/10.1111/j.1467-9450.2006.00513.x

Pearlman, L. A., & Curtois, C. A. (2005). Clinical applications of the attachment framework: relational treatment of complex trauma. *Journal of Traumatic Stress, 18*(5), 449–459. https://doi.org/10.1002/jts.20052

Ruff, S. C., Jones, C. L., & Clausen, J. M. (2019). A descriptive analysis of long-term treatment with adolescent-aged foster youth. *Journal of Child and Adolescent Trauma, 12*, 331–340. https://doi.org/10.1007/s40653-018-0233-9

Webster, L., & Hackett, R. (2011). An exploratory investigation of the relationships among representation security, disorganization, and behavior in maltreated children. In J. Solomon & C. George (Eds.) *Disorganized attachment and caregiving*, (pp. 292–317). Guilford Press.

van der Kolk, B. (2005). Developmental trauma disorder: Toward a rational diagnosis for children with complex trauma histories. *Psychiatric Annals, 39*, 5–26. https://doi.org/10.3928/00485713-20050501-06

Van Niewwenhove, K., & Meganck, R. (2019). Interpersonal features in complex trauma etiology, consequences, and treatment: A literature review. *Journal of Aggression, Maltreatment, and Trauma, 28*(8), 903–928. https://doi.org/10.1080/10926771.2017.1405316

13 Using the Adult Attachment Projective Picture System in pediatric health psychology

Parental gatekeeping and attachment trauma in an adolescent and his donor father

Marie Leblond, Marie-Julie Béliveau, and Marie Achille

Adolescents who receive a kidney transplant and their parents typically benefit from psychosocial support as part of standard care in recognition of the emotionally charged dimensions of this life-changing experience. Psychological interventions usually target reactions to receiving a foreign organ and managing post-operative demands (medication adherence, regular medical visits), with surprisingly little consideration for the profound relational implications of transplantation. Yet parents play a central role in supporting their child throughout the illness trajectory and sometimes even act as the donor. When a parent donates a kidney, it is considered a remarkable gesture and, adolescents tend to describe their overall experience in positive terms (Tong et al., 2008). But reactions may be more nuanced when a kidney is received from a parent during this complex developmental stage that involves building a separate and achieved identity and requires exploration and engagement (Erikson, 1968; Marcia, 1966). Indeed, research suggests the latter two are often lacking in adolescents who received a kidney transplant compared to healthy teenagers (Lugasi et al., 2013).

The purpose of this chapter is to examine the role of attachment when the adolescent's kidney donor is a parent. Attachment security plays an important role in facilitating adolescents' exploration of their sense of self and identity (Kerpelman & Pittman, 2018). Considering that parental reactions to diagnosis impact parent-child attachment in pediatric contexts (Oppenheim et al., 2009; Shah et al., 2011), attachment is worth documenting to better inform the care provided to adolescents with a kidney transplant. However, the role of the parent-child relationship in this context has yet to be examined. To this end, the Adult Attachment Projective Picture System (AAP, George & West, 2012), which allows direct access to adolescents' internal attachment representations, may be a particularly useful tool to access unconscious attachment

DOI: 10.4324/9781003215431-17

representations that impact identity formation in these youth. Used in combination with the AAP, the parent's Reaction to Diagnosis Interview (RDI; Pianta & Marvin, 1993) is likely to provide valuable information on the parental experience and its impact on attachment.

We describe here the case of a young adult male who received a kidney from his father when he was a teenager. This dyad was part of a larger qualitative study of adolescent kidney recipients, some of whom had received their kidneys from a parent (Leblond et al., 2020). The larger study explored the impact of donation on the parent-child relationship and identity formation. Father to son pediatric donation is rare; mothers donate more often than fathers for both medical and socioeconomic reasons (Jeswani, 2021; Rota-Musoll et al., 2021). As such, we considered this case study a particularly rich source of novel information.

Adolescence, attachment, and chronic disease

The process of attachment has been described as malleable across life in both the theoretical and empirical literature (Negrini, 2016). In early writings, the mother was considered the primary attachment figure, but there is increased attention to the role of fathers (Cowan & Cowan, 2019; Fagan et al., 2014). During adolescence, relationships with attachment figures can either facilitate or hinder the development of important competencies such as autonomy, independence, and the capacity to develop and maintain fulfilling relationships that are required for successful adult life (Allen & Tan, 2016). Adolescents are driven by a profound desire for independence and exploration and the goal during this period is to find a healthy balance between attachment behaviors (e.g., seeking proximity to attachment figures) and exploration (e.g., exploring new interests; Allen & Tan, 2016). Adolescents must feel security in attachment relationships to explore the world in their parents' absence.

The occurrence of an illness in children threatens the parent-child relationship and motivated research in the field of attachment in adolescents living with different chronic conditions (Pianta & Marvin, 1996). However, studies remain rare, and their results are contradictory. Some studies show no indication of more insecure attachment patterns among adolescents living with a health condition than healthy adolescents (Goldberg et al., 1990). Others show a higher proportion of insecure attachment patterns in adolescents living with a chronic condition (Berant et al., 2008; Goldberg et al., 1995). No study to date has examined adolescent attachment in the context of chronic kidney disease or kidney transplant. The numerous developmental disruptions associated with pediatric kidney disease and treatment (i.e., frequent hospitalizations, dialysis) and the unique role parents can play when they act as donors make attachment research in this area particularly relevant.

Chronic kidney diseases

Chronic kidney diseases can result from multiple conditions. When kidneys no longer function adequately, patients reach what is called end-stage kidney disease and start dialysis. Dialysis typically involves spending several hours connected to a machine in a dialysis center, two to three times per week. For young patients, this inevitably impacts school attendance as well as social and recreational involvement; for parents, it impacts all aspects of daily life. Dialysis in adolescents with end-stage kidney disease can last anywhere from a week to several years depending on the stage of the disease and characteristics of the child (Kasiske et al., 2010). It involves undergoing invasive procedures that have an impact on physical integrity and can induce distressing negative reactions, which may be experienced as even more distressing when a supportive attachment figure is unavailable.

Kidney transplantation is the only alternative when dialysis is no longer sufficient. While the transplant can be performed either from a cadaveric or living donor source, living donation is associated with better health outcomes (Nunes-Carneiro et al., 2019). In the context of pediatric kidney transplantation, a parent often volunteers to be the donor for their child. Kidney transplant considerably enhances health and life expectancy; however, it requires lifelong adherence to a regimen of immunosuppressive medication, and a patient may need more than one transplant throughout their life. Receiving a transplant during adolescence impacts quality of life, identity development, and parent-child relationships (Leblond et al., 2020).

Illness and parental experience

For most parents, initial exposure to diagnosis and illness occurs during early infancy and sometimes even during pregnancy. Finding out about the diagnosis is often a brutal and disruptive experience, marked by concerns over the children's condition, the realization of its implications, and, eventually, of the treatment involved. This initial period following diagnosis has aptly been described as traumatic (Pianta et al., 1996). Life as it had been hoped for rapidly changes into a shocking reality punctuated by setbacks, feelings of insecurity, stress, and fear (Akre & Suris, 2014).

According to Bowlby (1988), parents associate finding out about their children's diagnosis with a sense of loss and grief akin to losing someone through death. Responses include shock, denial, guilt, anger, and for most, eventually, acceptance or resolution (Pianta & Marvin, 1993). Parents who lack a sense of resolution are less likely to be available to soothe their children in distressing situations or behave in ways that foster the development of a secure attachment. Resolution status predicts parents' progression in dealing with their children's diagnosis and on the likelihood that they will be sensitive and flexible parents (Shah et al., 2011; Wachtel et Carter, 2008). It is therefore important to take into consideration parental experiences to fully understand adolescents' developmental experience in this context.

The case assessments

The AAP gives access to internalized attachment representations and the free-response format is a less confronting assessment method than a semi-structured interview. Often adolescents and parents claim to have a strong bond to defend against a conscious acknowledgment of negative feelings. The AAP gives access to the unconscious and internal realities of youth who are not always comfortable revealing all aspects of the parent-child relationship.

The RDI is an evidence-based assessment interview that reveals parents' progress in coming to terms with their children's condition (Pianta et Marvin, 1993). We selected it to describe the parent's dyadic experience and resolution status. The RDI includes a series of questions that evoke the parent's emotions and beliefs about the diagnosis, the child's condition, and reactions to events following the diagnosis. It is used in clinical research with populations presenting a range of health conditions, such as cerebral palsy (Schuengel et al., 2009) and autism (Yirmiya et al., 2015). Results from studies using the RDI confirmed that parents experience a sense of loss in reaction to illness and that resolution of the diagnosis is essential for the parents to be available to respond to their children's emotional needs and promote security in their attachment relationship (Oppenheim et al., 2009). This case study will present the father's responses to the RDI to provide a comprehensive description of the relational context within which the participant adolescent's attachment developed.

Adrian: A case study

Adrian's interview

Adrian is a young adult who is an only child. He lives with both parents in the province of Quebec, Canada. He received a kidney from his father when he was in his mid-teens. According to his medical history, his parents found out during his first weeks of life that only one of his kidneys was functioning, and poorly so. He spent most of his childhood and early adolescence being hospitalized repeatedly, sometimes for a few months at a time. He also suffered from conditions caused by his renal insufficiency, including urologic problems and chronic pain. Different specialists have been involved in his care at different times throughout his life.

Adrian was asked to describe his early years during an interview. He said he felt stressed when he experienced new symptoms and had to go to the hospital. He underwent several invasive procedures and painful lumbar punctures. Until his transplant, he had a catheter three hours per night, which precluded him from taking part in several social activities. Yet Adrian was resilient. Although he could not engage in many activities before the transplant, he described himself as a sports-oriented person as he was able to compete in ping pong tournaments.

Adrian described his relationship with his donor parent as open and supportive and marked by good communication. He did not consider his father overprotective but said he wished for more autonomy and independence. He said his father was frightened by situations that require autonomy such as letting him drive a car or go to a party. He felt he had to take excellent care of his condition to honor his father's gesture and he considered it crucial to take his medication daily. Lapsing into non-adherence could result in losing the graft, which he said would make him feel guilty.

Adrian said he knew from an early age that the day would come when one of his parents would be the donor. He remembered that after the transplant, he talked about the kidney as belonging to his father. He estimated it took him six months before he was able to consider the kidney his own. He said his father was helpful in this respect when he corrected him by saying "it is your kidney now."

Adrian's AAP

Adrian was classified as Unresolved; his main organizing (i.e., regulating) defense was deactivation. His AAP stories also showed defensive cognitive disconnection, indicating some underlying confusion and distress about attachment situations and affect. Adrian portrayed attachment relationships as functional; there was no evidence of attachment figures acting as a haven of safety in the alone stories or sensitive or mutual enjoyment synchrony in the dyadic stories. Six stories had segregated systems markers revealing self-representations as feeling empty and isolated, helpless, afraid of being abandoned, and a spectral dissolution of reality. Adrian showed a repertoire of containment strategies, including the capacity to act and internalized secure base (regulation with agency). Three stories, however, were Unresolved. Excerpts from his narrative are presented based on the following four themes: (1) emptiness and isolation, (2) failed protection by parental figures, (3) fear of death, and (4) fear of abandonment.

Emptiness

One theme throughout Adrian's AAP was feelings of emptiness and having to wait passively for an outcome when faced with a difficult situation. These elements are evident, for example, in his Window story.[1]

It's a girl, she comes home from *school* and she's	Deactivate
waiting for her parents. She's hungry and wants	Disconnect
to eat supper but the parents haven't come home.	
They're working. She is *bored* and she *thinks* it is	Disconnect
awfully long but then the parents arrive and she's	Agency: internalized
like, <u>I'm hungry</u>. They make supper and they eat late	secure base →
because they arrive late. She looks outside and feels	action
bored and *annoyed,* she asks herself, when are they	Disconnect
going to come? (Anything else?) It looks *empty,* it	Trauma
looks like an *empty* room.	Trauma

Confronted with the alone self as the first AAP stimulus, Adrian de-scribes the trauma of feeling isolated while waiting for parents to arrive (empty). Just starting the AAP task, Adrian demonstrates a capacity for agency; both the internalized secure base (the girl thinks) and the capac-ity to act reveal his representational capacity for agency. The girl thinks (internalized secure base) which leads to productive action (tells parents she is hungry) once the parents return. At least in response to the first probe to Adrian's attachment system, he demonstrates that he has the resources to wait in the face of trauma.

Failed protection by parental figures

Failed protection is the core of attachment dysregulation (George & Sol-omon, 2008; Solomon & George, 1996). Adult figures are sometimes absent altogether in Adrian's stories. When they are present, he describes them as feeling overwhelmed; the child is a burden, and they do not help the child. His responses to Bed and Corner demonstrate failed protec-tion. Here is his Bed story[2]:

This story describes Adrian's (child) internal experience at bedtime as a separation from the parent and he is afraid to be left alone. The narra-

The boy doesn't want to so he says, "I'm not tired, I'm	
not tired." He does not want to sleep, but the mother	
leaves him in his room and closes the door to try to get	
him to sleep. The boy is not happy with that, he can't	
sleep because he is *scared.* It is dark, and the mother is	Segregated system
angry because he does not want to go to sleep. (Next?)	Disconnect
He stays in bed but does not fall asleep because it is	
dark, and he doesn't like being in the dark alone. He's	
scared and the mother is not happy with her child	Segregated system
because he's *angry* at her and that's it.	Disconnect

tive demonstrates how Adrian and his attachment figure dance around the fact that he is frightened. The boy does not tell his mother directly and the mother either does not know or does not notice. The result is disconnected anger; the boy and his mother are angry at each other but for different reasons. The mother is angry because the boy will not go to sleep and the boy is angry because his mother leaves and does not protect him. Adrian is left alone and dysregulated.

Here is Adrian's Corner story[3]:

The beginning of the story indicates that Adrian is a bit disrupted by what he considers an odd image before he settles into the story. The projected self

This one is odd. I see that it is a small boy in a corner but this one is odd (silence). I don't know, it is a small boy in his corner being reprimanded. No no no that's not it, his parents are	
arguing and he doesn't like it, he does not want to see it, and he	Disconnect
does not want to hear anything and he's not well, and he's sad.	
His parents are *angry* at each other and he's **forced to see that**	Disconnect
because he's stuck there. Then one parent leaves and he's crying.	Trauma
I always end my stories on a sad note, don't I? I can come up with a happy ending. They will reconcile and it ends well.	

(boy) is rendered helpless by his parents' anger (arguing). The self is a small boy who is stuck, portraying an image of being powerless and trapped witnessing something he does not want to be a part of and for which he has no agency to change. The story ending demonstrates Adrian's conscious struggle against his parents' protective failure. He decides to tell a different ending, but he can only focus on parental reconciliation. We see that their reconciliation does not extend to the boy; nobody takes care of him. The story is Unresolved, and Adrian remains distressed and dysregulated.

Dealing with the concept of death

Adrian's questions about life and death are frequent and his stories tend to be dramatic and paralyzing. He often left the stories without a clear ending, overwhelmed by the internal conflict between hope for recovery and fear of dying. The story characters facing a traumatic situation are vulnerable, sad, and distressed. This theme was evident in Adrian's Bed and Corner stories above. It is also evident in response to a medical emergency in Ambulance.[4]

This narrative shows that Adrian is terrified by not knowing if an emergency medical situation will end in life or death. Notice that

There is one of his parents that had something like a heart attack and he's **freaking out** because he *doesn't know what*	Trauma,
to do, he *doesn't know what's going to happen* to his parent	Disconnect
so he's crying and he's sad. Then he could go to the hospital	Traumatic
with his grandma. It ends that *he either **dies** or he stays*	ambivalence
alive and he's ok. One or the other. They are **scared** because	Trauma
they *don't know* what's going to happen so they're	Disconnect
freaking out.	Trauma

the situation is so distressing that Adrian cannot assign an identity to the "boy" character; he is referred to by impersonal pronouns (e.g., he). The proposed remedy to this situation makes logical sense. Go to the hospital and find out if the grandfather died. Note though that nobody takes care of the child's fear, once again evidencing the theme of failed protection. There is no relationship synchrony. The grandmother (an attachment figure) neither comforts nor explains to the child what is going on. The story is Unresolved, and Adrian remains dysregulated.

Abandonment

Feelings of abandonment compound Adrian's representations of the helpless self and parental failed protection. The Bench story describes Adrian's feelings of utter abandonment.[5]

The Bench scene activates Adrian's feelings of helplessness (stuck, no way of getting out) with images of abandonment (orphanage). Adrian

Looks like a little boy living in an *orphanage* because there are *walls* behind and he looks *stuck* there. He's	Trauma
sad because he *does not have parents* and he would like to *escape.* He is in the *orphanage* since he was small, he never was anywhere else, and he would like to have a	Trauma
family. He goes to *sleep* in his bed and the next day it is	Deactivate
the same thing. Or maybe some parents could come and	Failed attempt
adopt him. He feels he's not lucky and that there is *no*	at connection
way of getting out.	Trauma

describes himself as isolated (wall) and not having a family. His attempt to deactivate (sleep) these intense feelings fails because, as he tells us, every day is the same. His situation never changes. He tells us that there is no escape.

The parent donor and his resolution of the diagnosis

Adrian's father is a construction worker in his mid-forties. The donation took place four years before the RDI. His father described that the first four years of Adrian's life were the most difficult for himself and his wife. He did not remember many details except a sense that they were unconscious during that period and their fear that their son was dying. Adrian's good moments during childhood did not offset the fact that the father felt he always had to prepare for the next challenge. Adrian always surprised the doctors, showing symptoms no one had ever encountered before, which left his father hypervigilant and in a constant state of alert. He and his wife made friends with other parents on the unit, which helped them feel supported by people who understood their feelings. The support group, however, did not effectively assuage the father's fears.

The RDI showed that Adrian's father was unresolved regarding his son's diagnosis. He said his first reaction was being frightened that Adrian might die. He explained that he had difficulty letting go of this thought and remained in a state of heightened alertness for years. This fear of death persisted even though he understood that the parent-donor transplant would have positive effects on Adrian's health and quality of life.

The father's narrative during the interview showed the degree to which he defended against his reaction to the diagnosis with avoidance of feelings. He denied reactions to the diagnosis, such as sadness, guilt, and injustice, yet these emotions continued to influence his everyday life. They likely continued to preclude him from achieving resolution of the diagnosis. The influence of these emotions could be seen in the father's behavior, visibly avoiding tension, experiencing confusion, and being overprotective. The interview raised the question of how Adrian's father was able to support, hold, and care for the emotional experience of his teenager through sickness and how this may have precluded his son from regulating intense emotions of helplessness, fear, and even abandonment when facing pain, invasive medical procedures, and hospitalizations.

Implications for psychological care

The results of the AAP and RDI can be useful for clinicians and health carers in creating a treatment plan. For Adrian, we would suggest individual therapy as the first line of treatment given the impact of attachment relationships on the psychosocial development of adolescents. His feelings of joy and gratitude at receiving a kidney expressed in his interview did not negate his conscious and unconscious emotions associated with attachment trauma revealed in the AAP. Moreover, his father's difficulty in coping with the diagnosis and avoidance of feelings made it more likely that Adrian will develop similar ways of coping and continue to be dysregulated when facing intense distress as an adult. Individual therapy could help him work through his experience with the illness and his relationships with his parents. Because he may feel a certain pressure from the father's emphasis on being positive, individual therapy provides a safe space to address personal issues with authenticity and develop feelings of control over his life.

Complimentary group therapy could help with Adrian's feelings of isolation by being with adolescents who have gone through similar experiences. A group setting could also be a good avenue to explore identity development, what it is like to receive a transplant from a parent, and how separation-individuation processes can be made more difficult by this experience.

Dyadic therapy sessions could help Adrian and his father address their relationship, taking into consideration the donation and their trauma in reaction to the illness. The objective would be to address the relationship, adversity, and emotional experience of both members of the dyad to foster adequate separation-individuation. The father and son relationship could also be supported by the therapist encouraging exploration of painful emotional experiences followed by sensitive responsiveness to gradually reduce the use of defensive exclusion.

Distressing situations are also experienced by the non-donor parent. Because chronic kidney disease in children often appears at a very young age and because attachment processes take root in the first years of life, it is necessary for those involved in the care of children with a chronic condition to provide services that are attuned to this reality to prevent future difficulties. Parents with sick children must mourn the life they imagined. Following diagnosis, the family receives emotional support from the medical team and access to a psychologist if needed, but the latter is not systematically offered. We believe that couple's therapy for these parents could help them face and sort out the many emotions experienced through the course of the illness and should be part of standard care. This intervention could be delivered according to a timeline that is sensitive to important points throughout the illness trajectory (e.g., resolving the diagnosis, deciding who will act as a donor, preparing for surgery, and after). Especially during the critical early years for the development of attachment, parents should be actively guided on the importance of sensitive responsiveness and successful protection.

Finally, to adequately support the child and his parents, health practitioners would likely benefit from being trained to become knowledgeable in attachment theory (see Chapter 1). This knowledge could enable staff and carers to recognize, for example, that children withholding the expression of attachment needs is not an indication of effective coping. Informed health practitioners could help facilitate children's access to attachment figures able to soothe and regulate high emotional and attachment needs when activated.

Conclusion

The case presented in this chapter illustrates the specific contribution of the AAP to deepen our understanding of the psychological and relational impact of living with chronic kidney disease and suggests that, despite this life-changing intervention, deep-seated fears persist well beyond the transplantation. Adolescents with a kidney transplant are a unique and small population; neither the adolescents' attachment nor the parent-donors' perspective were previously studied. Children's attachment patterns are influenced by their parents' capacity to resolve the diagnosis (Pianta & Marvin, 1993), and the threat to their children's life is an "assault" to the parents' caregiving system (George & Solomon, 2008). As we might expect, a chronic life-endangering condition threatens attachment security, presumably because of the exposure and challenges both the children and their parents must endure. For Adrian, the AAP made it possible to document the important difference between what he disclosed in his interview and his internalized attachment representations. Fears of abandonment, distress over the possibility of injury or death, and attachment figures' failures to protect him were not revealed during his interview. Adrian's internal emotional reality was quite different from what he portrayed externally, and the deactivation defense uncovered during the AAP was his attempt at self-protection from consciously grappling with attachment trauma and difficult emotions (Bowlby, 1980; George & West, 2012). The AAP demonstrated that his defenses failed. Adrian's attachment status was Unresolved and similarly, his father's response to his son's diagnosis was Unresolved.

Most adolescents who participated in our original study had insecure attachment representations, regardless of whether the parent was the donor. When faced with a threat to psychological or physical integrity, parents were distressed and had difficulty helping children regulate their emotions. Adrian's case was consistent with prior research that showed an Unresolved pattern in an adolescent is associated with the presence of challenging situations during infancy as well as a lack of security in the relationship between the child and his parent (Aikins et al., 2009). We can hypothesize that some of the AAP's pictures triggered trauma in Adrian, including flashbacks of his illness as a child and of the transplant. Attachment research would suggest the trauma was reinforced by his father's assault to caregiving, resulting in his inability to resolve the diagnosis and the behaviors that resulted, such as avoidance, overprotection, confusion, and fear (George & Solomon, 2008). In other words, unintegrated emotions associated with memories of the past and the father's caregiving representation and behavior are revealed in Adrian's stories, with themes of danger, failed protection, abandonment, injury, life, and death.

We have little information about the path to security for adolescents with kidney transplants. They may have received support from parents who were able to regulate more flexibly around the shock of and distress from their children's life-threatening illness. For Adrian's father, being the donor did not suffice to soothe the injustice or the helplessness he felt in reaction to his son's disease. Adrian's father showed indications that he still resorted to more rigid defense mechanisms and a goal-orientated coping style that likely precluded him from fully recognizing both his and his son's emotional experiences in reaction to the disease.

In summary, the combined use of the AAP and RDI in the context of this father-to-son kidney donation allowed access to underlying dimensions of their experience that offers a more nuanced and complex picture than could have been accessed through standard interviews or questionnaires. The emergent knowledge suggests the importance of monitoring attachment representations and diagnosis resolution to inform the development of care better suited to the parent-child dynamic.

This knowledge would be very valuable to help foster the conditions necessary for the development of secure attachment and autonomy of adolescents who face life-threatening conditions.

Acknowledgments

The first author received a doctoral research grant from the Kidney Foundation of Canada for this research. Special thanks are due to those who participated in this project and to all researchers who, with their knowledge, helped in making this manuscript sensitive and true to the experience of the participants. We also wish to thank Dr. Tom Blydt Hansen from Vancouver Children's Hospital and Dr. Marie-José Clermont from CHU Sainte-Justine, without them the project could not have been feasible.

Notes

1 Italics = defenses; bold = trauma; underline = capacity to act
2 Italics = defenses
3 Italics = defenses; bold = trauma
4 Italics = defenses; bold = trauma
5 Italics = defenses; bold = trauma

References

Aikins, J. W., Howes, C., & Hamilton, C. (2009). Attachment stability and the emergence of unresolved attachment during adolescence. *Attachment and Human Development, 11*(5), 491-512. https://doi.org/ 10.1080/ 14616730903017019

Akre, C., & Suris, J.-C. (2014). From controlling to letting go: What are the psychosocial needs of parents of adolescents with a chronic illness? *Health Education Research, 29*(5), 764–772. https://doi.org/10.1093/her/cyu040

Allen, J. P., & Tan, J. S. (2016). The multiple facets of attachment in adolescence. In J. Cassidy & P. R. Shaver (Eds.), *Handbook of attachment: Theory, research and clinical applications* (3rd ed., pp. 399–415). Guilford Press.

Berant, E., Mikulincer, M., & Shaver, P. R. (2008). Mothers' attachment style, their mental health, and their children's emotional vulnerabilities: A 7-year study of children with congenital heart disease. *Journal of Personality, 76*(1), 31–66. https://doi/pdf/10.1111/j.1467-6494.2007.00479.x

Goldberg, S., Gotowiec, A., & Simmons, R. J. (1995). Infant-mother attachment and behavior problems in healthy and chronically ill preschoolers. *Development and Psychopathology, 7*(2), 267–282. https://doi.org/10.1017/ S0954579400006490

Goldberg, S., Washington, J., Morris, P., Fischer-Fay, A., & Simmons, R. J. (1990). Early diagnosed chronic illness and mother-child relationships in the first two years. *The Canadian Journal of Psychiatry, 35*(9), 726–733.

Pianta, R. C., & Marvin, R. (1993). Manual for classification of the reaction to diagnosis interview [Unpublished manuscript]. University of Virginia, Charlottesville.

Pianta, R. C., Marvin, R. S., Britner, P. A., & Borowitz, K. C. (1996). Mothers' resolution of their children's diagnosis: Organized patterns of caregiving representations. *Infant Mental Health Journal, 17*(3), 239–256. https://doi.org/10.1002/(SICI)1097-0355(199623)17:3<239::AID-IMHJ4>3.0.CO;2-J

Shah, P. E., Clements, M., & Poehlmann, J. (2011). Maternal resolution of grief after preterm birth: implications for infant attachment security. *Pediatrics, 127*, 284–292. https://doi.org/10.1542/peds.2010-1080

Wachtel, K., & Carter, A. S. (2008). Reaction to diagnosis and parenting styles among mothers of young children with ASDs. *Autism, 12*, 575–594. https://doi.org/10.1177/1362361308094505

Yirmiya, N., Seidman, I., Koren-Karie, N., Oppenheim, D., & Dolev, S. (2015). Stability and change in resolution of diagnosis among parents of children with autism spectrum disorder: Child and parental contributions. *Development and Psychopathology, 27*(4), 1045–1057. https//doi.org/10.1017/S095457941500067X

14 Dismissive and blind to attachment distress

The AAP unravels a diagnostic puzzle

Rex Collins

Psychologists and psychiatrists often send their clients for assessment to provide external systematic evaluations and analysis to address clients' problems. This chapter describes the challenging case of a 17-year-old client referred to psychiatry for a medication review following an earlier diagnosis of a depressive disorder. The client had not attended school in the past year and had become increasingly withdrawn. He described episodes of depersonalization and derealization, along with sleep difficulties and intense anxiety. Interviews with his parents failed to determine any observable trauma or other adverse childhood events that would explain these symptoms apart from a prolonged period of enuresis. The psychiatrist noted that the client reported experiencing synesthesia, "seeing" sounds as colors. The client also expressed the view that numbers had "personalities." "Two is my friend; six is my enemy." Some sensory sensitivities were also noted. The psychiatrist, having observed an apparent episode of thought blocking during the interview with the client, became concerned that his withdrawal possibly presaged a potential psychotic break and a possible future diagnosis of schizophrenia. Consequently, the psychiatrist referred him for a comprehensive psychological assessment to shed light on his reality testing and his thought processes and assist in better understanding this troubled young man.

The chapter discussion shows how the AAP helped the assessor unravel this young client's Failed Mourning for attachment trauma, characterized by creating a defensive wall against memories of failed protection, compounded by lingering feelings of shame and derealization. The chapter also demonstrates how integrating AAP results with other testing data, particularly those of the Rorschach, resulted in a rich understanding of this young man's psychopathology, and lead to a helpful sharing of the findings with the client, the psychiatrist, and the parents. The process by which the assessor arrived at his findings is described in detail.

Mathew: A case study

The young client, Matthew, had been described by parents as a "happy, outgoing, and extraverted kid" until around grade 8 (age 13) at which

DOI: 10.4324/9781003215431-18

time he appeared to become more introverted and depressed. He had been designated as intellectually gifted and an excellent student up until grade 12, when he stopped attending class and became increasingly withdrawn. He is the youngest child with two older brothers, one of whom has been diagnosed with Autism Spectrum Disorder. His parents are successful academics.

In interview, Matthew, a fair haired 17-year-old adolescent of medium height, is easy to engage; his eye contact is good, and he relates appropriately to the assessor. He is notably candid in sharing his worries and his self-experience. There is a sense that he sees the assessment as an opportunity to unburden himself and to seek to understand what is happening to him.

He speaks of his sleep difficulties. He has trouble falling asleep. He often wakes in the night from bad dreams and nightmares, and reports having great difficulty distinguishing his dreams from reality. He tells of a dream in which he was responsible for "the deaths of hundreds of people" and was terrified until he slowly realized that it was, in fact, a dream. After these dreams, he will fall into a sleep so deep that he cannot be roused. Naturally, during the time he was attending school, his oversleeping would result in his being frequently late for class.

He speaks of his anxieties. Walking into class late made him feel "constantly observed – being seen in a vulnerable moment." While he could sometimes manage the sense of being "judged" by his classmates, he was more troubled by what the teacher might think of him. He would occasionally avoid this situation by going to a nearby park and staying there for the entire day. This tension was not confined to this past year at school. He remarks as well, "I was very unhappy in elementary school, but it felt more like regular unhappiness."

During the period of this evaluation, Matthew could not make the journey to school "unless I'm feeling physically and mentally all right – it's hard to cross that threshold." He described the transition from the warmth of his bed and the privacy of his room to "a building full of students is a freaky thing, a different mode, a very weird difference."

Matthew hesitates before speaking of "another element" in his anxiety. He says, "I get so, so ... horribly stressed thinking about objectivity, the realness of things, and how people think about morals." He is concerned about the "social web," that is, the cultural norms, values, and morality that are the basis of a society, lamenting that "objectivity is never possible." How could he consider himself a "good person" if there were no objective measures of this? Yet even if the social web is somehow suspect, the alternative is a kind of empty void where nothing has meaning. Matthew says of these musings, "it feeds into the loneliness thing and the anxiety. I have an anxious, terrified mind about how cold and dark the world is and how alone I am." He emphasizes that his worries about objectivity are the most troubling aspects of his anxiety, and laments, "I get flustered and anxious when I can't articulate things properly." This statement is as if to say that, despite his efforts, he has not been able to convey to the assessor the nature and depth of his existential anxieties.

He goes on, "also I'm really stressed at just being in my body." He describes the experience of fixing his gaze on his fingers and thinking how "gross" his fingers and his face are. In a subsequent interview, Matthew describes an episode of anorexia, noting that

> I've always had a neurotic attitude to, like, having a body, and thinking about weight. It makes me feel gross or whatever. A couple of years ago I think I had a BMI that was at an unhealthy level, but I still disliked the way my body looked. Even though I felt dizzy and lightheaded, I needed to find some way to lose weight.

At the end of the first interview, challenging questions arise in the mind of the assessor. Matthew presents and engages well, is intelligent, and is articulate in his description of his difficulties (although he's not quite sure of this himself). There is a psychotic feel to his hallucinatory dream experiences, as well as an autistic feel to his overriding preoccupation with the nature of objectivity. And what of his attachment issues? The contrast between his account of his unhappiness in his elementary school years and the narrative provided by his parents could suggest a dismissive attitude on their part to his attachment needs. There is also his stated fear of being all alone in the world. What light might psychological testing shed on this complicated and troubling picture?

Psychological testing

Four tests comprised the test battery employed to attempt to elucidate the complex picture this young man presented. The Millon Adolescent Clinical Inventory (MACI), a self-report inventory, was selected as a means by which Matthew could convey perhaps more thoroughly his perceptions of his issues. The Rorschach and the Differential Diagnostic Technique (DDT) could shed light on his reality testing and thought processes. The Adult Attachment Projective Picture System (AAP) would provide a measure of his state of mind regarding attachment, the interpersonal matrix of his disturbing symptomatology.

Matthew's MACI profile suggested a possible diagnosis of Generalized Anxiety Disorder and Dysthymic Disorder, with Schizoid and Depressive personality traits with Self Defeating and Avoidant features. Scales reflecting Identity Diffusion and Self-Devaluation were also elevated, with high scores on Introversion and Inhibition. The test showed an emerging picture of a sad, cautious, insecure young man who had little hope that others might provide him support and nurturance when he needed it. Overall, the profile confirmed the findings of the clinical interview and Matthew's reported history.

A follow-up question concerning his endorsement of an item reflecting suicidal ideation revealed that Matthew did experience thoughts of self-harm from time to time saying, "It's not that abnormal to think about." When younger, he had entertained ideas of suicide by jumping off a tall building. He felt this would give him the exhilarating experience of flying, but added, wryly, "it wouldn't be good if you changed your mind halfway down."

The Rorschach and DDT results confirmed that Matthew had problems with reality testing and thought processes. His reality testing as measured by the Rorschach indicated a degree of impairment bordering on the psychotic, and his thinking was at times illogical and incoherent. For example, Matthew responded to Card VI with the following:

> This part's a fiery sort of sun in the background. Unfortunately, it would make this part like an ice cream from an ice cream stand. With the sun, there's fiery flames coming out of it, a dramatic representation of the sun and its heat, but if you go to an ice cream shop, the ice cream's shaped like Sponge Bob. The nature of the runniness of the ink material looks like it's melting with the hot sun in the background.

His response is perceptually distorted and indicative of tangential, confabulated, and illogical thinking. These results were confirmed by a close examination of his DDT protocol.

However, it was a striking pair of responses to Card VII of the Rorschach that particularly caught the assessor's attention. On examining the card, Matthew responded "Kind of looks like two women who are joined at the hips. Instead of legs they just have the other person's body coming out and they're just having a conversation." This percept was followed by "some kind of like, I don't know, a rock formation standing in the water but it's falling over." These consecutive percepts appeared to encapsulate a central notion of the early psychoanalytic theories regarding the nature and precipitants of autistic withdrawal and self-stimulating behaviors – both characteristic of autistic children. That is to say that the infant's experience of a premature rupture (real or imagined) in the symbiotic bond with the caregiver results in a kind of sudden terrifying separateness where the immature body/self may be experienced as falling, fragmenting, or dissolving. From this perspective, autistic anxieties are considerably more frightening than anxieties related to being judged or criticized, or being rejected or abandoned since they relate to a terror of the dissolution of the body/self. Matthew's stated preoccupation with the reality of objectivity and his statement "I have an anxious, terrified mind about how cold and dark the world is and how alone I am" seems to resonate with this view of the nature of autistic anxieties. His fantasy to fly when commenting on his suicidal ideation may be seen as a primitive defense against the fear of falling and fragmenting.

At this stage of the review of the test results, the picture of Matthew that is emerging is that of a young man whose seemingly neurotic level of functioning overlays what might be called an "autistic core," or in Joshua Durban's (2020) view an "autisto-psychotic core." Durban notes

> The child on the autisto-psychotic spectrum manifests a mixture of paranoid-schizoid anxieties and other less well-differentiated anxieties-of-being such as: liquefying, spilling out, dissolving, having no skin or skin full of holes, losing parts of the body or falling into bits, freezing, burning, losing a sense of time and space, and existing in a bi-dimensional world. The autistic child experiences mainly the latter.
>
> (p. 94)

Thinking about Matthew from this perspective, and the idea that "autistic anxieties" manifest out of a premature rupture with the caregiver, the question of Matthew's attachment – his pattern of relating to others – weighs heavy on the mind. What is the interpersonal matrix within which these troubling symptoms manifest themselves? How might an examination of his AAP protocol add to and deepen the understanding of Matthew's symptomatology that would be helpful to him and his treating professionals? Understanding Matthew's attachment seems imperative to understanding him, his anxieties, his fears, and how to best help him.

The AAP

Matthew's AAP classification is Dismissing, Failed Mourning, a result strongly suggestive of a failure to address a trauma or perhaps multiple traumas in his life. (See Chapter 2 for an in-depth discussion of Failed Mourning and the AAP.) How can one reconcile this finding with the parents' view that no notable trauma had occurred during Matthew's life to date?

His protocol is noteworthy in the intensity of trauma it revealed. Three of his alone stories have segregated systems trauma markers in the response – Window, Bench, and Corner; trauma was also evident in Bed, a story he told to the dyadic "mother" scene. Attachment dysregulation is also depicted in Ambulance and Cemetery; however, the story elements do not reach the level associated with traumatic fear. It was significant, therefore, that Matthew's overall response to the AAP showed that by far attachment situations terrify Matthew and that he must continually manage potential collapse throughout the AAP. His AAP also contains derealization markers (dereal, evidence of distressed disengagement from reality or depersonalization), which emerge when the projected self is alone in Window and Corner. It is also significant that the bulk of the derealization markers show up in his response to Corner, the final picture of the series, which depicts a child in a corner with arms outstretched as if to ward something off. Matthew's Corner story[1]:

This kid, standing in a corner um that's displaying an aversion to something, showing that he finds something *gross* or displeasing, doesn't want it anywhere near.	Derealized shame state
He looks like a ***vulnerable position 'cause he's sort of backed up in a corner***, but it doesn't look anything too serious, 'cause he's making a sort of cartoonish and	Trauma
animated cliché movement of what looks like *disgust* to me. So it just looks like *disgust* (laugh) with something, no matter how, whether more literal sort of sensory *disgust* or, whatever. He's got his hands outstretched as if, you know, there's something in particular he wants	Derealized shame state
to <u>keep away from him</u>. He's got his hear turned away,	Agency: action
like *I can't even look at you*. Well, I don't know, maybe whoever he's with might say he's very rude and he might get in trouble.	Derealized shame state

   There is a pervasive and palpable sense of trauma-related disgust and shame in Matthew's story, heightened by the fact that the boy is helpless in a "vulnerable position." Indeed, there are five derealization markers related to things being disgusting or "gross." Depersonalization imagery often contains elements that are more easily seen as related to episodes reported in other patients' accounts of their out of body experiences. What the disgust and shame markers have in common with these experiences, however, is an implicit wish and impulse to be invisible, to be somehow outside of one's disgusting and shameful body. Here the assessor's thoughts return to Matthew's report in his interview that "I'm really stressed at just being in my body," his reported brush with an eating disorder, and to how he would fix his gaze on his fingers thinking how "gross" they and his face were. Several questions emerge. Is the boy in the story disgusted at himself? At something he's done? At someone else? At someone else's reaction? ("I can't even look at you.") How might this apparent self-view be related to trauma and its lingering effects? And what might be the relative contributions of a possible "autistic" trauma as suggested by his Rorschach response, and a more cumulative trauma, such as his chronic enuresis, resulting in feeling disgusting and ashamed?
   Following a review of the psychological tests, Matthew is questioned about his earlier chronic enuresis. At first, he shrugs it off. It was just something he and the family learned to live with, a view that is consistent with the dismissing features of his AAP protocol. After relating

several behavioral interventions that were tried over the years, Matthew pauses. He recalls how disappointed both he and his parents would feel when, following a seemingly successful intervention, the enuresis would return. It is hard to escape the notion that, despite Matthew's dismissal of this persistent embarrassing experience, he has lived with an ongoing sense of shame and the feeling that his body was letting him down. Likely as well was his sense of his parents' displeasure, distaste, perhaps disgust as he continued to wet the bed. ("I can't even look at you.")

Theater of the body

From the results of the assessment, it seems evident that a distorted relationship with his body is the underlying percept associated with Matthew's current difficulties with his school attendance, and feelings of vulnerability. The integrated findings of the Rorschach and the AAP add depth to this understanding by elucidating what might underlie this young man's distress and discomfort with his body and the world around him.

In conceptualizing the contribution of trauma to his current psychopathology, it might be useful to think of a distinction between what might be called "big T" and "little t" trauma. Big T trauma is a serious injury, debilitating illness, or loss of a significant person in one's life. "Little t" trauma reflects cumulative and ongoing unprotected micro-assaults on one's sense of safety, self, self-worth, and self-esteem that result from chronic attachment figure failed protection (George & Solomon, 2008). George and West (2012) demonstrate that failed protection in response to a barrage of assaults must be conceived as attachment trauma and evidence shows that these experiences can be as debilitating as big T trauma. Much of Matthew's chronic fear may be, therefore, conceived as little t trauma in response to his parents' failed protection and lack of sensitivity to be aware of his vulnerability to shame.

Matthew's striking Rorschach response described earlier strongly suggests he experienced what Frances Tustin (1972) would call a "premature psychological birth," a deep rupture in the neonate's early sense of "weness" that is often accompanied by primitive fears of the body falling, fragmenting, or dissolving. This was an experience Matthew was to attest to during the feedback session. His evident intellectual strengths and his relatively adequate, if superficial, social skills would preclude a diagnosis of Autism Spectrum Disorder. However, the test results did suggest the presence of what might be called an "autistic core" in his overall personality functioning. This could perhaps be considered a "big T" trauma, one, however, which can easily escape the notice of even the most dedicated parent. Likely, Matthew's constitutional givens of intelligence and motility, along with an average expectable parenting environment, contributed to his following what, on the surface, seemed to be a reasonably normal path until adolescence, when the tasks of separating and individuating from the parents (Blos, 1967) and assuming ownership of the sexual body (Laufer & Laufer, 1995) become paramount. Viewing Matthew's problems as essentially those of school refusal together with some depressive affect and anxiety is not adequate to explain the complexity of his troubles.

At this juncture, a close review of his AAP protocol yields important information in further unraveling this complexity. As noted above, Matthew's response to Corner involves a child who is in "a vulnerable position, 'cause he's sort of backed up into a corner." The child is "displaying an aversion to something, showing that he, uh, finds something gross, doesn't want it anywhere near." Later, "he's got his head turned away, like, I can't even look at this, I can't even look at you." It's not hard to link this story to Matthew's experience of chronic enuresis and the shame he experiences around it. In particular, his statement "I can't even look at you" suggests a wish to turn away from seeing a possible look of dismay, disapproval, or even disgust on a parent's face. A clear behavioral indication of a retreat into deep shame.

Shame, according to Smith (2009), creates an "unwanted separation from the caregiver." A close reading of Matthew's response to Bed, the fifth picture in the series depicting a child in bed reaching their arms out toward an adult figure (seen by most as the mother) seated at the other end of the bed, seems to delineate his possible reaction to this unwanted experience. Matthew's Bed story[2]:

So it looks like sort of a mother and her sort of young son's room...he's in bed, she's sitting at the end of his bed. It looks like * *he's reaching out for a hug from her*, but the strange part is she appears to be gripping her wrist.	* Attachment signal
Maybe she injured her wrist or something and it seems like she's gripping her wrist and sort of, at least in the moment *ignoring her son's extent*. I'm going to say maybe somehow accidentally the son injured his mother's wrist, and so she's sitting there sort of massaging her wrist and	Deactivate – reject
he feels bad so *he's going in to give her a hug*. The son feels he's accidentally done something to hurt his mother. He feels really bad, he wants to be reassured that everything's alright, and she still loves him. The mother seems pretty	Child repairs to stay connected
unbothered, she doesn't think it's too big a deal and it's probably going to be okay. I'm *hoping* this mother accepts	Deactivate Disconnect
her son's request for a hug, and that he goes to bed and he feels alright and her wrist gets better (laughs) and, um, *we find out that it's a happy mother-son relationship*.	Disconnect

In this story, the son has somehow accidentally damaged the mother (nighttime bedwetting is typically referred to as an "accident"); the mother's psychological wound (her disappointment with Matthew's chronic enuresis?) has become a physical wound, and the son must make some reparation ("he's going in to give her a hug") to maintain a connection to her. It is perhaps notable that Matthew's mother had reported to the psychiatrist that he had recently become particularly attuned to her emotional state. Matthew's body has not only let him down but has also threatened his relationship with his primary caregiver.

Matthew's Window story, a picture of a young girl looking out of a picture window, captures the ensuing emptiness and isolation that he has described in interview during the assessment, and his longing for, yet his estrangement and distance from the world. Matthew's Window story:

Okay... (deep breath)... so it looks like a little girl looking out a window. The inside of her house is a little bit *blank*	Trauma
and plain and maybe she lives in a *boring* and *closed in*	Disconnect
sheltered lifestyle, and she is *looking out at the outside*	
world and thinking about what it would be like if she was	Dereal
more free. I suppose it looks like a window in a living room or something, so I would imagine she walked into her living room and then walked up to the window and is now standing at the said window. Maybe she can't go outside, and because of that she feels that it's been, she feels	
choked. Maybe *she has an idealized sense of what it's like*	Trauma
to go outside and see things and be in the fresh air, and	Dereal
maybe she's longing for that. ... Well, um ... (laughs) you	
know, I would *hope* for her sake that she gets to go outside,	Disconnect
but maybe she doesn't. It's *hard to judge what she's doing*	
or *what she's supposed to be doing* ... um, like... (laughs).	Disconnect

We note that the "inside of the house looks a little bit blank" likely reflecting Matthew's internal world. "She lives a boring and closed in sheltered lifestyle and she is looking out at the outside world." This latter phrase smacks of the surreal and is coded as a derealization marker. There is a sense that his feelings of emptiness are so profound that he must mentally flee (dissociate) from his reality into a surreal imagined "space" of freedom from his pain and distress. And even though "an idealized sense of what it's like to be outside" beckons, it is likely not without its real dangers and its unreal quality. Recall Matthew's comment that "being in a building full of students is a freaky thing, a different mode, a very weird difference." Matthew's story, which is his first response to the AAP task, suggests he lives in a state of suspended animation, "choked" and constricted, like the girl, who seems to somehow float mindlessly in the story. "She walked into her living room and then walked up to the window, and is now standing at said window." There is an aimlessness, a lack of intent, motivation, or agency, and there is no sense of her immediate history. Where was she before walking into the living room? What motivated her to go there? Although, "I would hope for her sake that she gets to go outside, but maybe she doesn't. It's hard to judge what she's supposed to be doing, um... (voice trails off and he laughs)." Matthew is choked in what Steiner (1993) calls a "psychic retreat," that is to say, too anxious to regress in order to mourn his failed protection, or to progress in the direction of successfully negotiating the developmental process of adolescence. If only, as he wishes for the girl, he could be "more free." Free from what? Free to do what? The overall assessment would suggest a wish to be free of shame, as well as a wish to be free of the more primitive fears of bodily fragmentation and falling.

The passivity and lack of agency in this story prompt questions about Matthew's capacity to exercise appropriate healthy aggression and assertiveness. Where is his anger at being shamed? At himself? At his parents for their possible dismissal of his attachment needs? At their "disgust" at him? Whereas guilt can leave open avenues for reparation, shame leaves the self (and the body) weakened, flawed, and unworthy of asserting itself in the world. Any anger or rage at the person or persons shaming one is then buried deep in the psyche and, when this happens, the individual is robbed (or robs him- or her-self) of the vitality and energy that fuels making an impact on one's world. (There is growing evidence (C. George, Personal Communication, October 28, 2021) that the repression and disavowal of anger toward the caregiver for their failed protection is characteristic of those individuals whose AAP protocols are coded as Dismissing, Failed Mourning.)

Matthew's striking response to the Rorschach Card IV is relevant here and offers a way toward understanding this dimension of Matthew's struggles.

> Some big vaguely humanoid creature standing above you. You're looking up at it. Its arms have been chopped off and it's looking angrily down at you. (Inquiry) Huge Titan-like Japanese monster, something out of Japanese anime, once again looks insect influenced. The head of an insect and the tail hanging down and you're looking up at it. You see those areas, holes that are just dripping, looking down at you. The head is looking down, the arms are cut off and it's looking down. (As if?) In your head you could imagine you've cut the big monster's arms off but now it's angry with you and you're singled out and it's going to crush you like that and you're thinking you made a mistake.

Here, the dominating and frightening figure (a parent?) is "looking angrily down at you," seemingly because "in your head, you could imagine you've cut the big monster's arms off." There are parallels here to the "wounded" mother in Matthew's Bed story, although in his Rorschach response the damage to the monster's body is not an "accident" and reflects a more intense murderous rage. Engaging in conflict with the monster however causes intense fears of even more murderous retaliation ("It's going to crush you like that") and so such fantasies must be rigidly repressed, although they may emerge in dreams. (Recall Matthew described a dream/hallucination where he was responsible for the deaths of hundreds of people.) The roots of his passivity, then, can be hypothesized as arising from his pervasive sense of shame, as well as a need to repress anger and healthy aggression. It is also perhaps noteworthy that the damage to the body reflected in his Rorschach response adds another dimension to the autistic-like fears of bodily fragmentation.

The picture of Matthew that has emerged from the results of the psychological tests is, as noted, far more complex than that of school refusal by a depressed and anxious teenager. It is evident that underlying Matthew's current difficulties and feelings of vulnerability is a distorted relationship with his body, intense shame, and profound difficulties with his experience and appropriate expression of healthy anger and aggression. As well, the striking evidence of derealization in Matthew's AAP protocol, and his reports of experiencing depersonalization and derealization, the sense of leaving one's body and observing it from a distance, the implicit wish to be invisible, suggest viewing these episodes as primitive ways of distancing himself from his endangered and shameful body. Recall also his fantasy of committing suicide by jumping off a tall building and experiencing a sense of exhilaration – another defense against his deeper fears of fragmentation. Matthew also remains choked by his repressed and disavowed rage toward his attachment figures, unable to assert himself appropriately in the world, or to emerge from his autistic "shell," which speaks directly to the self-imposed constriction ("choked" like the girl in Window) that happens when called upon to take action and engage with the world around him.

Conclusion

The results of the assessment, particularly the intersection of the AAP and the Rorschach, provide a generative hypothesis with which to understand the complexity of this troubled young man's psychopathology. If credence is given to the first Rorschach response described, then Matthew experienced a "premature psychological birth" as suggested by Tustin. Since no physical reasons could be found for his chronic enuresis, it can be hypothesized that his ongoing bedwetting arose from this deep, unconscious anxiety, which was recalcitrant to any behavioral interventions, and beyond the conscious awareness of both Matthew and his parents. Its persistence resulted in interactions with his mother that, for Matthew, became a deep source of shame and threatened his attachment to her. Now, at the developmental stage where Matthew's task is to separate and individuate from both his internal and external objects and to take ownership of his own (sexually mature) body, he is plagued by a deep and primitive ambivalence for both his state of mind concerning attachment and to the integrity of his body. Profound inhibition of his need to assert himself in the world, coupled with a deep-seated fear of retaliation if he does, has left Matthew stuck in what he seems to consider an impossible bind. Addressing these issues will require of his therapist an attunement to the differing depths of his difficulties – to the complex layer of shame that compromises his security and that overlays his "autistic core."

The coding of his AAP protocol is apt. However, it seems, at this point, Matthew is not fully aware of what it is he has to mourn. The assessment pattern shows that what Matthew has to mourn is little t trauma intrinsically related to attachment figure failed protection. Matthew will need to come to the painful acknowledgement that his parents were unable to be sufficiently aware of the depth of his fears, his emptiness, and his shame to provide him with the level of support he was unable to reach out for, or even clearly articulate. He will need therapeutic support as he moves through the grief cycle of his deep sadness about this, and his anger at the misattunement of his parents to his deeper needs.

It is to be hoped, then, that the report of the lengthy psychological assessment will have provided to the mental health professional entrusted to his care some kind of "road map," a direction informed by the contributions of both the Rorschach and the AAP, that will show the way toward Matthew's attaining a stronger and more resilient sense of self and a capacity to engage in the world in a more authentic and assertive way.

Notes

1 Italics = defenses; bold = trauma; underline = capacity to act
2 Italics = defenses; bold = trauma

References

Blos, P. (1967). The second individuation process of adolescence. *The Psychoanalytic Study of the Child*, 22(1), 162–186. https//doi.org/10.1080/00797308. 1967.11822595

Durban, J. (2020). From chaos to Caravaggio: Technical considerations in the psychoanalysis of autisto-psychotic states in relation to sensory-perceptual fragmentation. *Journal of Child Psychotherapy*, 46(1), 90–104. https://doi.org/10.1080/0075417X.2020.1730422

George, C., & Solomon, J. (2008). The caregiving system: A behavioral systems approach to parenting. In J. Cassidy & P. R. Shaver (Eds.), *Handbook of attachment: Theory, research, and clinical applications* (2nd ed., pp. 833–856). Guilford Press.

George, C., &West, M. (2012). *The adult attachment projective picture System: Attachment theory and assessment in adults*. Guilford Press.

Laufer, E., & Laufer, M. (1995). *Adolescence and developmental breakdown: A psychoanalytic view*. Karnac Books.

Smith, A. (2009). Distinguishing the holistic context of the inferiority-superiority strivings: Contributions of attachment and traumatic shame studies. *Journal of Individual Psychology*, 65(3), 241–263.

Steiner, J. (1993). *Psychic retreats. The new library of psychoanalysis*. Routledge.

Tustin, F. (1972). *Autism and childhood psychosis*. Hogarth.

15 The role of the Adult Attachment Projective Picture System in treating childhood obesity

Claudia Mazzeschi, Elisa Delvecchio, Livia Buratta, Daniela Di Riso, Silvia Salcuni, and Adriana Lis

Childhood obesity is a significant problem in our world today, affecting a child's health and their emotional well-being and relationships with peers and family (Farpour-Lambert et al., 2015). The drastic increase in overweight youths in the United States and Europe over the last 30 years has led psychologists and other health professionals to examine what might be contributing to this complex and detrimental issue (e.g., Harrison et al., 2011; Serra-Majem & Bautista-Castaño, 2013). Psychological components are considered crucial: preadolescents and adolescents with overweight/obesity and disordered eating, with the high prevalence of girls, often carry significant emotional problems and experience profound distress with peers and family (Evans et al., 2017). Moreover, specific family features and structures, an abnormal familial climate, and a dysfunctional parent-child relationship contribute to obesity and weight problems (Berge et al., 2014; Mazzeschi et al., 2013). This chapter illustrates using the AAP to elucidate the relationship foundation of obesity in the case of a young girl referred for weight problems in a center for obesity treatment using a family-based approach.

Attachment is a recent addition as a "new" dimension to understanding obesity because of its power to grasp the relational aspect of human functioning in terms of an internal representation of attachment (internal working model; e.g., Lacasa et al., 2015). Bowlby (1980) viewed the internal working model of attachment as the precipitate of the early relationships and attachment experiences characterizing the inner representational world of the self. In this sense, attachment is the expression of an emotional nucleus of felt security and perceived protection from danger at the presence, real or internalized, of an attachment figure and relationship. The unconscious mental representation of attachment, developed in the early and ongoing parent-child relationship, serves as a self-regulating mechanism and an emotion-regulating process that promotes self-regulation in those first and later in other relationships. Attachment theory offers a developmental perspective when considering the emergence of weight gain, eating disorder symptoms, and their association (Gander et al., 2015).

DOI: 10.4324/9781003215431-19

An increasing number of obesity studies use an attachment theory framework (Fiese et al., 2012; Frankel et al., 2012). These studies highlight the role of young children's insecure attachment and low parental responsiveness as the connection to the onset of weight problems later in life (Anderson et al., 2012; Anderson & Whitaker, 2011; Coutinho et al., 2020). They also discuss the role of negative regulation strategies and emotion-feeding pressure practices by insecure parents (Bost et al., 2014).

Interest in the different contributions of both parents has also increased. Insecurity with the father is significantly associated with more concerns about eating and higher report of subjective and objective binge eating; however, the mother relationship seems more strongly associated with children's eating pathology and weight status (e.g., Goossens et al., 2012). These studies support the importance of including an extensive evaluation of the mental representation of attachment (Tasca et al., 2011) in the clinical assessment of obesity and its developmental risks.

Assessing the unconscious mental representation of attachment is crucial to grasp the internal processes and dynamics of the self-regulative mechanism. All the above studies used self-report measures, which only elicit conscious appraisals. The use of free-response narratives and performance-based instruments evokes unconscious mental representation. Assessments like the *Adult Attachment Projective Picture System* (AAP) provide a comprehensive window into the emotional strategies, correlations, and consequences of individual differences in attachment system functioning and the strategies individuals developed to cope with the anxiety aroused by the tasks. In short, these assessments overcome biases such as social desirability that can affect self-report results (George & West, 2012; Mazzeschi et al., 2014).

Evaluating attachment patterns helps assess the relative weight/role of parental and individual factors contributing to the clinical condition in the complex association between obesity and risk for eating disorders in adolescence using a family-based approach. In this period of life, parental and family context factors play an essential role (Fiese, 1997). The parent-child relationship in pre-adolescence predicts vulnerability for psychopathology in adolescence (Mezulis et al., 2006). A family-based approach is considered the gold standard for treating obesity in childhood (Skelton et al., 2012). Within this context, evaluating attachment provides incremental validity for the clinical assessment of this complex and heterogeneous syndrome by identifying the unique and interrelated role of the self-regulating mechanisms for each family member.

Our collaborative assessment lens: Integrating the AAP into assessment

Using the above framework, the CURIAMo[1] developed a family-based model for assessing and treating overweight-obesity in youths (see Mazzeschi et al., 2014, for a comprehensive description). The most substantial effects in treating the psychological features of overweight-obesity require including the parents as intervention targets. The psychological portion of this program is characterized by counseling centered on each family's needs. The program uses established psychometric psychological measures that demonstrate their characteristics, strengths, and weaknesses, such as psychological risk factors, family functioning, parenting alliance and practices, attachment when needed.

The psychological work begins with an assessment phase to evaluate the child's and parents' risk factors associated with overweight-obesity. Assessment is followed by psychoeducational groups of parents or adolescents and two follow-up sessions. Psychotherapy is also recommended if the assessment results suggest it is needed.

The assessment phase follows a collaborative therapeutic assessment approach (Finn, 2007) to maximize parents and youth involvement. Involving parents is considered crucial for the intervention, expanding treatment success rate (Gilles et al., 2008). The AAP is administered in this phase. Youths and their parents also completed self-report measures (described below). Parent self-report measures provide better predictors of child outcome than physical measures (e.g., body mass index). Moreover, parental functioning influences the course of the intervention (Zeller et al., 2007).

A case study: Claudia and her parents

Claudia, age 15, was referred for treatment at the CURIAMo by her parents because of her eating practices. She is the only child of an intact family. Physically, Claudia appears plump and a little obese. Claudia and her parents were interviewed separately during the assessment phase.

Claudia says she is sometimes anxious about her "body shape and weight" and would like to be slimmer to become a hostess. For this reason, she tries to follow her mother's suggestion about diet, but at the same time, she finds it very difficult to resist food. She complains about parental control over what and how much she eats. Their approaches to her eating and her life are different. Her mom is calm and detached; her father is anxious and uncontrolled. Claudia complains that her father is also very controlling about her school achievement. Being at the top of her class is not enough for her father.

Claudia's peer relationships are uneven. She is very proud that she made many international friends on their family summer cruise because she was able to speak different languages. She says that she has some good friends that talk and go out together. However, she said it was not easy when she was younger because her peers teased her about her weight. She describes a pool party where some classmates made fun of Claudia in her swimsuit, calling her a "whale." Although she found herself crying in her bedroom, she was very detached when describing this incident and concluded that now "it is all ok."

Claudia's parents' appearance and their approach to Claudia's problem with food are quite different. Her mother has a slim, slender build. Her mother emphasizes the importance of healthy foods, which she tries to prepare and share with Claudia. Her examples stress how Claudia is happy to follow her mother's rules about food, school, and other aspects of her life. She describes their relationship as good and affectionate.

In contrast, her father looks overweight. He says that Claudia was always like the way she is now; she was a little "plump" from when she was a child, and "she has always eaten with gusto, ...as me..." (smiles as he indicates his round belly). He tries to follow the mother's diets but says sometimes it is challenging for him to have small portions. He regrets his mother's ways of dealing with food. Sunday lunch at his mother's home always has plenty of food on the table. The family milieu is to eat with "gusto," not controlling how much or what you eat. Claudia's father describes their relationship with anxiety and ambivalence. He focuses on the crucial achievements in every aspect of Claudia's life and how he can fly out of control when Claudia is not "doing her best."

Claudia's parents agree that she is growing well, although they also remember a specific episode when one of her primary schoolmates made fun of her because of her body shape. They were happy that this child did not go to Claudia's high school, concluding that "It is all forgotten." They agreed that the most important was that Claudia is at the top of her class and has good friendships.

Clinical assessments

Clinical assessments began with the body mass index (BMI) assessed when they first arrived at the clinic. Claudia had a BMI of 30.2, indicating low-level obesity. The mother, age 38, had a BMI of 25.39, and the father, age 41, had a BMI of 29.7. (BMI assessed on arrival to the clinic.)

The family also completed a set of self-report measures. Her parents completed the Child Feeding Questionnaire (Birch et al., 2001; Buratta et al., 2021), which assesses the parents' perceptions of their own and their children's weight status, concerns about weight, and feeding practices. Both parents engaged in restrictive feeding practices, taking excessive control of Claudia's food intake. They paid exaggerated attention to Claudia avoiding junk or unhealthy foods. Claudia completed the Spence Child Anxiety Scale (Spence, 1997) and the Body Uneasiness Test (Cuzzolaro et al., 2006). The Child Anxiety Scale assesses anxiety symptoms. Claudia's results showed clinical levels of panic agoraphobia and social phobia and near-clinical levels of fear of physical injury and obsessive-compulsive symptoms. She specified in particular worries about her body image. Her Body Uneasiness Test results showed significant body dissatisfaction (worries about physical appearance) and a fear of becoming fat with compulsive monitoring of her body appearance. She was especially dissatisfied with her body parts, such as her legs and buttocks, and her physiological reactions, such as blushing.

AAP results

The AAP was administered individually to Claudia and her parents during the assessment phase. We begin with the results of Claudia's AAP.

Claudia's classification is Dismissing, Failed Mourning (see Chapter 4). This representation indicates that Claudia has experienced attachment distress as traumatic (i.e., attachment figure failed protection, George & Solomon, 2008). She attempts to regulate by armoring herself and detaching from her parents' intense affect. The AAP showed weak agency of self – no thoughtfulness and the capacity to act in only two of the four alone stories). Her stories showed that she does not feel connected to others, and she views attachment figures as distant and removed or not present.

Claudia's view of parental absence and alternative regulation strategies is demonstrated in Ambulance.[2]

There is someone here (she indicates the stretcher)? ...	
So they are carrying away someone in the ambulance	
... he/she is looking outside the window.... probably	
he/she knows the person the *paramedics* are taking	Deactivate
away, probably he/she is *worry* and the other figure is	Disconnect
tranquilizing him. and... That the person who is carried	Deactivate
away felt ill and so they have called the ambulance	
which is arrived... ...after this person was able to	
tranquilize him/her... they will go to the hospital to	Deactivate
know how he is ...Beh ... him or her, let's say is *worry*	Disconnect
is probably *frightened*, instead the other figure feels	Segregated system
compassion, but according to me *she is not really*	Deactivate
involved, she is only there in that moment to try to	
tranquilize the other person.	Deactivate

Notice how a social role figure (paramedic) takes care of the ill person by taking this person to the hospital. The two central figures in the picture (a woman and a boy), however, are unidentified; the projected self (boy) is labeled "he/she" and the potential caring adult that is identified in most responses around the world as a grandmother is reduced to "the other person." Claudia's disconnected worry and fear in response to a medical emergency are evident in her story. The other person, described as "not really involved" (deactivated by distance), tranquilizes those emotions (deactivate). This story shows how Claudia can name worry and fear but is prevented from showing them.

The Corner picture activates attachment with the greatest intensity (Buchheim et al., 2008). Claudia's response reveals her distress as traumatizing (see Chapter 4).[3]

Here he is *frightened*...he puts his hands up, so he is	Trauma
frightened, he defends himself from someone, he is *cornered*	Trauma
...so he tried to *escape* before to be *blocked*...and....before	Trauma
... *I don't know* ...someone wants to *hurt* him ... and so	Trauma, Disconnect
later *I do not know* what will happen. *Fear* maybe.... *I*	Trauma, Disconnect
don't know....I have really to create a story? Mm...Maybe	
it was night and he was going around alone, and a *criminal*	Trauma
had seen him, and his intentions were really bad. He tried to	
escape, but later *he was blocked* in this corner, and now *he*	Trauma
cannot do anything to defend. and.... How will it finish? If	Trauma
we are positive, he will be able to *escape,* or someone will	Trauma
see him and help him. Maybe a *policeman.*	Deactivate

Claudia shows us in this story how she is helpless (cornered), afraid, and desperate (needs to escape) she feels when she is feeling persecuted (criminal). She attempts to control her affective response first by trying to disconnect but finally deactivates. Her terror is so intense that she can name a social role figure (policemen) as coming to her assistance in this story. The story is void of attachment signals (i.e., communicating the need for care) and attachment figures.

In sum, Claudia's AAP shows that she walls off feelings of attachment distress and trauma, trying to segregate fear and helplessness (i.e., repress) from consciousness. The AAP, however, makes her trauma visible. This survival strategy indicates a very fragile state of mind. According to Bowlby (1980), Claudia is primed for dysregulation; she is a risk of plunging into an unresolved state of helplessness and despair should her deactivating defenses fail.

Her mother's AAP classification is Unresolved. This representation indicates that Claudia's mother becomes frightened and flooded by her attachment fears when confronted with situations that trigger feelings of being frightened or helpless. Some of these situations are residues from her childhood; other situations likely include her daughter's obesity (George & Solomon, 2008). Her mother's AAP shows poor agency; the projected self shows no expectation for comfort from attachment figures (haven of safety) or no capacity for integrative reflective thinking. The Corner story was the only time her mother showed the capacity for action, suggesting that only the most threatening attachment situation would elicit images of protective behavior. Claudia's mother becomes sentimental in her response to Bed, an image that portrays a mother and her child. She describes the situation as "affection, tenderness, need of cuddles" but cannot immediately act on this evaluation. The mother's response in Bed thereby fails to demonstrate sensitive caregiving (Ainsworth et al., 1978). Like Claudia, her mother's main regulating defense is deactivation; her defensive goal is to create distance in relationships and turn away from distress. The mother's AAP also evidences segregated systems. Her Ambulance story shows how attachment figures can regulate a frightened child with reassurance, which is then deactivated, as in Claudia's response. Bench and Cemetery, however, push Claudia's mother over the edge. She can neither exclude nor regulate feelings of being lost and desperate. Here we show Bench[4]:

This looks like *an athlete*. She *failed* a volleyball match (she	Deactivate
laughs), and now she is on the bench, **desperate** because	Trauma
she made a mistake ... I don't know in *the volley match*	Deactivate
or in an exhibition of an artistic gym, what she is feeling...	
I would like to say sadness again, *she is sorry*, maybe next	Disconnect
time things would be better. Then it can happen that she	
will go back to play, *hoping* to play better	Disconnect

This narrative demonstrates how the projected self's achievement failure activates desperation, negative self-evaluation (made a mistake), and disconnected regret (is sorry). The mother shows she has the will to make changes but fails to develop a strategy. She lives on hope. In the absence of agency, we see also that no attachment figures or others help her. She is desperate and utterly alone.

Claudia's father's AAP classification is also Unresolved. Like her mother, representation of the projected self alone fails to include images of comfort or integrative thinking. He does demonstrate, however, the capacity to act. When available in the dyadic pictures, he can see attachment relationships as providing comfort and consolation. Her father's main regulating defense is cognitive disconnection. Unlike the deactivation of his daughter and his wife, Claudia's father's main regulating defense is cognitive disconnection. He cannot entirely exclude distressing experience and affect; disconnection creates a fog or smokescreen so that he cannot identify sources of distress or how they are managed. He is preoccupied, ambivalent, and confused about attachment until responding to the last two AAP pictures, where he becomes dysregulated. Confronted with a "visit" to a past relationship in Cemetery and the potential threat of being alone and unprotected depicted in Corner are dysregulating. In Cemetery, the father shows his response to anger. Here is her father's Corner story:

Ah (he laughs) something else.... *fear?* Ah what happened	Trauma
before? *Maybe he had done something bad or he was*	Disconnect,
scolded... or he was hit. Ok. Later it could happen that//	Trauma
The re-pacification with the//...so there is not the other	
face, I do not see the other face... I see *fear*... this I see	Trauma
fear... to approach him. He does not want the contact. He is	Trauma
cornered, he was sent to the corner. I think that once one is	Trauma
fighting, then he tries to stop, no? ... to find a solution, **Fear**,	Disconnect
anger, **pain**, but **pain** maybe *I don't know* surely *fear* and	Trauma,
anger maybe... nothing more is coming in my mind.	Disconnect

Claudia's father is frightened, helpless, and preoccupied with what we must assume is attachment figure anger. He is so distressed that he "cannot see the other face," creating a representational fog that obscures this person's identity. Attachment trauma overwhelms his regulatory capacity.

Clinical considerations and conclusions

Claudia's parents referred her to CURIMo for a specific symptom: obesity. However, the CURIMo process incorporates a psychological approach to a child's problems and the family system. The AAP provided an added perspective to this complex situation.

Claudia is indeed a plump girl whose BMI indicates a low level of obesity. She is, however, also an adolescent where body awareness and social comparison are typical sources of angst. Her discomfort with her body was evident from her interview, including her goal to realize her ideal self and become a slim hostess. However, peer shaming about her weight began in childhood, suggesting that Claudia's problems were not simply normative adolescent worries. We see her deactivating defenses kicking in when she sloughs off the teasing by saying it was now all ok. Her self-report assessments showed her anxiety and body dissatisfaction. The AAP provided a deeper picture of Claudia's attempt to slough off her experiences, including demonstrating her dismissing representation of relationships and the traumatic level of her wounds and unavailability of her attachment figures.

We spoke with her about her test results during the restitution phase of treatment. The conversation was not so difficult. Her assessments demonstrated the convergence of conscious and unconscious awareness. She came to recognize that "underneath" she is not ok. One of the essential conversations was discussing her AAP results during this phase. The first point of discussion was how Claudia used dismissing defenses to distance herself from her emotions and regulate when they were about to overwhelm her. She acknowledged that "they are still in the back of my mind."

Dismissing attachment (the mature analog of child avoidant attachment) develops when the child knows that the parents are not available and reject their needs; dismissing individuals regulate by detaching themselves from parents. In Claudia's stories, we saw potential images of parents being replaced by other people, including social role figures. Being in a state of Failed Mourning, we know that trauma was in the back of her mind. She was frightened and helpless, and she could not envision attachment figure protection from her feelings or peer persecution. The next step for Claudia is that she needed to mourn. Following Bowlby (1980), Claudia needed to interrupt the cycle of unconscious deactivation of her fears and worries and begin to address them directly, bringing them out in the open for discussion and help.

The psychologist discussed this conundrum with Claudia, suggesting that she felt her parents had concentrated too much on obesity and controlling food and school. This discussion raised thoughts that perhaps Claudia would like to have her parents more connected with her feelings about her adolescence and her personal life. She agreed she would like to have support from them about issues not related to food. She did not understand why this was so difficult for them but had some idea that their problems sometimes blocked them from understanding she was asking for help.

The parents' interviews showed scarce awareness of their daughter's feelings; they were only oriented toward her physical symptoms and their achievement demands. Their demands did not always attune with Claudia's needs, such as problems with friends about which they seemed oblivious. The AAP showed the complexity of the parents' internal world. Both were unresolved and helpless; her mother was desperate, and her father was frightened. Neither of their regulating defense structures – deactivation for mother and disconnection for father – was working. Neither demonstrated the quality of agency, connections to others, or relationship synchrony that would be needed to respond to their sad and frightened daughter.

One of the strengths of the AAP is that it is not a biographical interview; therefore, it can detect segregated fear, pain, isolation, and helplessness that the parents either did not want to address or could not name. The parents also needed to mourn. Talking with them about their AAP results was not so easy because, being unresolved, they could be easily overwhelmed by the results. Overwhelmed, they could be flooded by their trauma and lose sight of the goal to provide Claudia with the protection and support that she needed to grow.

The psychologist started by talking about the difficulties of parenting an adolescent girl because of the changes that occur at this time. The psychologist underlined how the mother thought about the importance of regulating "healthy" food and how sometimes a parent can feel unprepared, lost, and even desperate when talking with a young adolescent. The discussion with Claudia's father addressed how an attempt to control her academic life was a response to shifting his attention away from more frightening thoughts, such as her daughter is a "whale." Both parents were supported to understand how underlying feelings of helplessness were crushing their efforts to be "good parents." Their concrete strategies to date were substitute ways to deal with Claudia's problem.

Studies have shown that parents' representations of their attachment relationships affect parenting (George & Solomon, 2008). The unresolved pattern lacks a coherent and unique strategy; parents with this pattern risk becoming deeply disturbed by their unresolved experiences and helpless to "see" and address their children's distress (George & Solomon, 2008). These parents are at risk for ineffective parenting behaviors, frequently observed in studies of parental and familial functioning of children and adolescents with obesity (Lehto et al., 2012; Sleddens et al., 2011). Claudia's parents' AAPs fit this picture, which put Claudia in the position to deactivate her traumatic distress and distance herself from her parents to find help elsewhere. Distancing helps her maintain a regulated attachment pattern but uses robust defenses with a waste of energy. No matter how hard Claudia tries, this approach is not a good way to face her problems or adolescent development.

These delicate and deep issues arise during the feedback phase of the consultation because the CURIAMo model stresses the importance of parent collaboration and their need to be involved in an obesity problem. Focusing only on weight loss without considering the concerning symptoms and signs described by Claudia would put the intervention at risk for failure. Attachment is crucial for its power to uncover the emotion-regulating processes affecting Claudia's family dynamics when addressing her problem. For this reason, her parents are recommended during feedback to continue their psychotherapy to work on the sources of their tenacious response to Claudia's weight. Her weight, combined with her parents' helplessness and unavailability, puts Claudia at risk for social isolation, irritability, difficulty concentrating, profound fear of gaining the lost weight back, and body image distortion. The feedback session stressed the importance of psychotherapy for Claudia to address her psychological suffering, or in Bowlby's words, to mourn. It was also vital for her to get help with her obesity using the lifestyle program offered by the CURIAMo clinic.

Notes

1 A university clinic with a multidisciplinary core located in Perugia, Italy.
2 Italics = defenses
3 Italics = defenses; bold = trauma
4 Italics = defenses; bold = trauma

References

Anderson, S. E., Gooze, R. A., Lemeshow, S., & Whitaker, R. C. (2012). Quality of early maternal-child relationship and risk of adolescent obesity. *Pediatrics*, 129(1), 132–140. https://doi.org/10.1542/peds.2011-0972

Anderson, S. E., & Whitaker, R. C. (2011). Attachment security and obesity in US preschool-aged children. *Archives of Pediatrics and Adolescent Medicine*, 165(3), 235–242. https://doi.org/10.1001/archpediatrics.2010.292

Ainsworth, M. D. S., Blehar, M., Waters, E., & Wall, S. (1978). *Patterns of attachment: A psychological study of the Strange Situation*. Erlbaum.

Berge, J. M., Rowley, S., Trofholz, A., Hanson, C., Rueter, M., MacLehose, R. F., & Neumark-Sztainer, D. (2014). Childhood obesity and interpersonal dynamics during family meals. *Pediatrics*, 134(5), 923–932. https://doi.org/10.1542/peds.2014-1936

Birch, L. L., Fisher, J. O., Grimm-Thomas, K., Markey, C. N., Sawyer, R., & Johnson, S. L. (2001). Confirmatory factor analysis of the child feeding questionnaire: A measure of parental attitudes, beliefs and practices about child feeding and obesity proneness. *Appetite, 36*(3), 201–210. https://doi.org/10.1006/appe.2001.0398

Bost, K. K., Wiley, A. R., Fiese, B., Hammons, A., McBride, B., & The STRONG KIDS Team. (2014). Associations between adult attachment style, emotion regulation, and preschool children's food consumption. *Journal of Developmental and Behavioral Pediatrics, 35*(1), 50–61. https://doi.org/10.1097/01.DBP.0000439103.29889.18

Bowlby, J. (1980). *Attachment and loss: Loss, sadness and depression* (Vol. 3). Basic Books.

Buchheim, A., Erk, S., George, C., Kächele, H., Kircher, T., Martius, P., Pokorny, D.,

Buratta, L., Delvecchio, E., Germani, A., & Mazzeschi, C. (2021). Parental feeding practices across child's weight status: Evidence of the Italian validation of the Child Feeding Questionnaire. *Public Health Nutrition, 24*(6), 1256–1264. https://doi.org/10.1017/S136898002000381X

Coutinho, V. M., Queiroga, B. A. M. de, & Souza, R. C. (2020). Attachment style in children with chronic diseases: A comprehensive review. *Revista Paulista De Pediatria, 38*, e2018308. https://doi.org/10.1590/1984-0462/2020/38/2018308

Cuzzolaro, M., Vetrone, G., Marano, G., & Garfinkel, P. E. (2006). The Body Uneasiness Test (BUT): Development and validation of a new body image assessment scale. *Eating and Weight Disorders: EWD, 11*(1), 1–13. https://doi.org/10.1007/BF03327738

Evans, E. H., Adamson, A. J., Basterfield, L., Le Couteur, A., Reilly, J. K., Reilly, J. J., & Parkinson, K. N. (2017). Risk factors for eating disorder symptoms at 12 years of age: A 6-year longitudinal cohort study. *Appetite, 108*, 12–20. https://doi.org/10.1016/j.appet.2016.09.005

Farpour-Lambert, N. J., Baker, J. L., Hassapidou, M., Holm, J. C., Nowicka, P., O''Malley, G., & Weiss, R. (2015). Childhood obesity is a chronic disease demanding specific health care—A position statement from the childhood obesity task force (COTF) of the European Association for the Study of Obesity (EASO). *Obesity Facts, 8*(5), 342–349. https://doi.org/10.1159/000441483

Fiese, B. H. (1997). Family context in pediatric psychology from a transactional perspective: Family rituals and stories as examples. *Journal of Pediatric Psychology, 22*(2), 183–196. https://doi.org/10.1093/jpepsy/22.2.183

Fiese, B. H., Hammons, A., & Grigsby-Toussaint, D. (2012). Family mealtimes: A contextual approach to understanding childhood obesity. *Economics and Human Biology, 10*(4), 365–374. https://doi.org/10.1016/j.ehb.2012.04.004

Finn, S. E. (2007). *In our clients' shoes: Theory and techniques of therapeutic assessment*. Routledge.

Frankel, L. A., Hughes, S. O., O'Connor, T. M., Power, T. G., Fisher, J. O., & Hazen, N. L. (2012). Parental influences on children's self-regulation of energy intake: Insights from developmental literature on emotion regulation. *Journal of Obesity, 2012*, e327259. https://doi.org/10.1155/2012/327259

Gander, M., Sevecke, K., & Buchheim, A. (2015). Eating disorders in adolescence: Attachment issues from a developmental perspective. *Frontiers in Psychology, 6*, 1136. https://doi.org/10.3389/fpsyg.2015.01136

George, C., & Solomon, J. (2008). The caregiving system: A behavioral systems approach to parenting. In J. Cassidy & P. R. Shaver (Eds.), *Handbook of attachment: Theory, research, and clinical applications* (2nd ed., pp. 833–856). Guilford Press.

George, C., & West, M. L. (2012). *The adult attachment projective picture system: Attachment theory and assessment in adults.* Guilford Press.

Goossens, L., Braet, C., Van Durme, K., Decaluwé, V., & Bosmans, G. (2012). The parent-child relationship as predictor of eating pathology and weight gain in preadolescents. *Journal of Clinical Child and Adolescent Psychology,* 41(4), 445–457. https://doi.org/10.1080/15374416.2012.660690

Harrison, K., Bost, K. K., McBride, B. A., Donovan, S. M., Grigsby-Toussaint, D. S., Kim, J., Liechty, J. M., Wiley, A., Teran-Garcia, M., & Jacobsohn, G. C. (2011). Toward a developmental conceptualization of contributors to overweight and obesity in childhood: The six-Cs model. *Child Development Perspectives,* 5(1), 50–58. https://doi.org/10.1111/j.1750-8606.2010.00150.x

Lacasa, F., Mitjavila, M., Ochoa, S., & Balluerka, N. (2015). The relationship between attachment styles and internalizing or externalizing symptoms in clinical and nonclinical adolescents. *Anales de Psicología (Annals of Psychology),* 31(2), 422–432. https://doi.org/10.6018/analesps.31.2.169711

Lehto, R., Ray, C., & Roos, E. (2012). Longitudinal associations between family characteristics and measures of childhood obesity. *International Journal of Public Health,* 57(3), 495–503. https://doi.org/10.1007/s00038-011-0281-5

Mazzeschi, C., Pazzagli, C., Laghezza, L., Battistini, D., Reginato, E., Perrone, C., Ranucci, C., Fatone, C., Pippi, R., Giaimo, M. D., Verrotti, A., De Giorgi, G., & De Feo, P. (2014). Description of the EUROBIS program: A combination of an epode community-based and a clinical care intervention to improve the lifestyles of children and adolescents with overweight or obesity. *BioMed Research International,* 2014, 546262. https://doi.org/10.1155/2014/546262

Mazzeschi, C., Pazzagli, C., Laghezza, L., De Giorgi, G., Reboldi, G., & De Feo, P. (2013). Parental alliance and family functioning in pediatric obesity from both parents' perspectives. *Journal of Developmental and Behavioral Pediatrics,* 34(8), 583–588. https://doi.org/10.1097/DBP.0b013e3182a50a89

Mazzeschi, C., Pazzagli, C., Laghezza, L., Radi, G., Battistini, D., & De Feo, P. (2014). The role of both parents' attachment pattern in understanding childhood obesity. *Frontiers in Psychology,* 5, 791. https://doi.org/10.3389/fpsyg.2014.00791

Mezulis, A. H., Hyde, J. S., & Abramson, L. Y. (2006). The developmental origins of cognitive vulnerability to depression: Temperament, parenting, and negative life events in childhood as contributors to negative cognitive style. *Developmental Psychology,* 42(6), 1012–1025. https://doi.org/10.1037/0012-1649.42.6.1012

Ruchsow, M., Spitzer, M., & Walter, H. (2008). Neural correlates of attachment dysregulation in borderline personality disorder using functional magnetic resonance imaging. *Psychiatry Research: Neuroimaging,* 163(3), 223–235. https://doi.org/10.1016/j.pscychresns.2007.07.001

Serra-Majem, L., & Bautista-Castaño, I. (2013). Etiology of obesity: Two "key issues" and other emerging factors. *Nutricion Hospitalaria,* 28(Suppl 5), 32–43. https://doi.org/10.3305/nh.2013.28.sup5.6916

Skelton, J. A., Buehler, C., Irby, M. B., & Grzywacz, J. G. (2012). Where are family theories in family-based obesity treatment?: Conceptualizing the study of families in pediatric weight management. *International Journal of Obesity, 36*(7), 891–900. https://doi.org/10.1038/ijo.2012.56

Sleddens, E. F. C., Gerards, S. M. P. L., Thijs, C., de Vries, N. K., & Kremers, S. P. J. (2011). General parenting, childhood overweight and obesity-inducing behaviors: A review. *International Journal of Pediatric Obesity, 6*(2–2), e12–27. https://doi.org/10.3109/17477166.2011.566339

Spence, S. H. (1997). Structure of anxiety symptoms among children: A confirmatory factor-analytic study. *Journal of Abnormal Psychology, 106*(2), 280–297. https://doi.org/10.1037//0021-843x.106.2.280

Tasca, G. A., Ritchie, K., & Balfour, L. (2011). Implications of attachment theory and research for the assessment and treatment of eating disorders. *Psychotherapy, 48*(3), 249–259. https://doi.org/10.1037/a0022423

WHO Consultation on Obesity (1999: Geneva, Switzerland), & World Health Organization. (2000). *Obesity: Preventing and managing the global epidemic: Report of a WHO consultation* (No. 894; WHO technical report series). World Health Organization. https://apps.who.int/iris/handle/10665/42330

Zeller, M. H., Reiter-Purtill, J., Modi, A. C., Gutzwiller, J., Vannatta, K., & Davies, W. H. (2007). Controlled study of critical parent and family factors in the obesigenic environment. *Obesity, 15*(1), 126–136. https://doi.org/10.1038/oby.2007.517

16 Attachment-informed assessment of adolescent conduct disorder

A case study

David Joubert

Externalizing behavior problems and delinquency are common reasons for referring adolescents to mental health or social service agencies, especially for boys (Steiner et al., 2007). It is generally recognized that adolescents presenting externalizing problems differ in terms of the severity of the misconduct, problem onset, presence of aggression toward others, level of social and cognitive impairments (e.g., deficits in moral reasoning), presence of comorbid internalizing problems, and callous-unemotional personality traits (Cardinale et al., 2018; Fragkaki et al., 2016; Gambin & Sharp, 2016; Song et al., 2016). These characteristics may, in many cases, be modifiable through appropriate rehabilitative intervention. Clinicians must nevertheless obtain a broad picture of psychological functioning to understand better the ontogeny of each individual's conduct problems (Piccirillo & Rodebaugh, 2019).

Attachment theory (Bowlby, 1979) proposes a theoretical framework that can account on a phenomenological level for some of the pervasive social and interpersonal difficulties associated with the more severe forms of externalizing problems (i.e., conduct disorder or psychopathy; Pasalich et al., 2012; Rosenstein & Horowitz, 1996). One of the main attachment theory contributions is that it allows for understanding personality functions and processes from a developmentally-based relational perspective (Mikulincer & Shaver, 2012). Early attachment relationships are considered one of the primary building blocks for personality development (Bowlby, 1982). Careful consideration of attachment organization may yield helpful information on the best ways for incorporating relational-interpersonal elements in treatment with this population. It may also provide insights into differential diagnosis, for instance, by helping account for specific characteristics that are central to the construct of juvenile psychopathy, such as callous-unemotional traits (van der Zouwen et al., 2018). In addition, processes of defensive exclusion associated with deactivation of the attachment behavioral system may facilitate proactive and instrumental forms of aggression.

In contrast, the relational enmeshment typical of preoccupied individuals may contribute to reactive-affective violence. By contrast, segregated system material (see Chapter 1) associated with Unresolved

DOI: 10.4324/9781003215431-20

attachment may lead to aggression accompanied by dissociation or other trauma reactions (Meloy, 1992; Taubner et al., 2013, 2016). This type of information is useful both from the perspective of risk assessment and therapeutic or case management. The chapter uses a case illustration to highlight the use of attachment information provided by the Adult Attachment Projective Picture System (AAP) in the assessment and subsequent case formulation of a young offender in a carceral setting.

Case study: John

John is a 16-year-old Caucasian male who was incarcerated in a facility for juvenile offenders at the time of the assessment. He was found guilty on charges of theft and reckless endangerment, for which he was given a sentence of 18 months. John was adopted at approximately 3 years of age by a stable family living in a rural setting. His mother left him under the state's care shortly after birth, presumably due to long-standing mental health and substance use issues. He exhibited hyperactive and distractible behavior during his formative years, but he was a lovable child who had no significant conduct problems by his parents' account. Risk factors associated with early life may include potential exposure to substances in utero, maternal history of mental health problems, and abuse or neglect from the custodial staff at the orphanage. However, none of these were ever officially confirmed.

Behavioral issues emerged in adolescence around 13 years of age. John's relationships with his parents and the school and community environment became more conflictual as he began to resent any supervision and control over his behavior. Behavioral issues including impulsivity, attention-seeking, lying, truancy, opposition, and minor delinquency (vandalism, theft) became increasingly prominent. Serious problems arose over time in the relationship between John and his parents as he became unwilling to accept any parental monitoring and supervision. His parents mentioned that while John can often make a good impression on others, this tends to quickly crumble as he "cannot tell the truth" and does not appear to care about the consequences of his actions on others. For instance, John mentioned bullying a weaker peer at school, conduct that he described as justified on the basis that the peer was "disgusting" and "weird" and was, therefore, "asking for" abuse. John's parents were dismayed at what they described as his capacity to deny wrongful behavior even when presented with evidence of it, such as video footage of him stealing.

John is never without his phone and spends a significant amount of time on social media. His parents are worried about what they described as "attention-seeking behavior" on his part, including making racist and misogynistic comments or engaging in aggressive "role-play scenarios" online. For instance, he posted a video of him kicking the family cat. He also has difficulty in his relationships with female authority figures, particularly his mother. His parents describe him as "obsessed with girls" he meets online. He has run away from home on several occasions to meet these teenage girls, at one point stealing the family vehicle. Once, he attempted to run over one of the young girl's family members after they told him to leave. He also falsely accused his father of physically abusing him after being picked up by the police when he ran away from home.

John's most recent offense that led to arrest occurred after his parents confiscated his phone after a period of excessive use. This transgression led to an intense argument, following which John managed to retrieve the phone from a safe, shut down the smoke detectors, and set fire to the bed on which his parents were sleeping. The father sustained burns on his hands, trying to extinguish the fire. John waited outside until the firefighters arrived. He was then taken under custody by the local police. A psychological assessment was requested approximately six months into the sentence. The custodial staff did not believe that John was engaged in rehabilitative efforts and was puzzled at his apparent lack of remorse for his wrongdoings, especially the injuries to his father's hands.

At the time of the assessment, John's parents were quite ambivalent about the possibility of having him back home. The notion that he may have entertained the thought of killing them was a severe blow to their relationship with John, as he had already made similar threats in the past, although never directly to them. Consequently, they were torn between concerns for his well-being and their safety. During the interview, John made it clear that he harbored deep resentment regarding his parents' supervision of his activities, believing that they have no right to take his property and should "mind their own business." He denied wanting to harm or kill his parents. Instead, his actions that night were reportedly done for "showing them he would not be pushed around." He also clarified that he should have stolen the family truck and driven away rather than waiting for the authorities to arrive. John readily acknowledges making threats to his parents and peers at school but denies planning on acting upon them. He could not describe either parent in terms of their personality or unique attributes, describing only the functional aspects of their relationship (e.g., taking him to sports, making his bed, cooking).

Since being institutionalized, John has shown a marginal level of adjustment to unit life and routine. He expresses little interest in rehabilitative activities and has been subjected to multiple disciplinary measures for minor rules violations. While not directly engaging in violent behavior, he does tend to provoke peers and then rely on staff intervention to avoid retaliation. In the school setting, he obtains marginal grades in most subjects, with areas of strength in Gym and History. While he recognizes the importance of education, he also reports that most of his teachers would describe him as disruptive in class. He sees himself as a "popular guy" who can easily influence others around him. When questioned about whether he has ever felt remorse for something he has done, John brought up setting the house on fire, clarifying that he did not want to hurt anybody and that if he could go back, he would not have done it and "screwed up his life." He denied ever having been depressed or upset. The parents also suggested this, who remarked that to their knowledge, he has never been sensitive to rejection and generally does not tend to express deep emotions.

Overview of psychological assessment results

The psychological assessment with John included a clinical interview and checklists completed by the parents, self-report questionnaires, and several implicit assessment methods. In order to better understand John's internal models of attachment relationships, the AAP – an implicit method of assessment – was used to assess his attachment pattern. The behavior checklists supported the presence of significant problems consisting of oppositional or defiant conduct, delinquency, hyperactivity, impulsivity, and inattention. Broadband self-report personality questionnaires (MMPI-A, MACI) emphasized deceitfulness and low tolerance to frustration, problems with impulse control, weak interpersonal relatedness, and lack of capacity for moral reasoning. It was noted that adolescents with similar profiles tend to appear self-sufficient, with little need for close emotional interactions with others. They are also poor candidates for traditional psychotherapy. Findings from implicit assessment methods (Rorschach, TAT) highlighted John's propensity for action over thinking and reflection, poorly developed representations of others, and lack of emotional investment in relationships. Strong tendencies toward impulsivity and egocentrism were also prominent.

John was also assessed using the Psychopathy Checklist – Youth Version (Forth et al., 2003). He obtained a score of 27/40, slightly below the cut-off value for a diagnosis of juvenile psychopathy. It was concluded that some aspects of John's psychological and social functioning were consistent with the callous-unemotional nature of psychopathy. In contrast, the extensive history of offenses typical of primary psychopaths was less evident. In this context, attachment assessment was mobilized to understand better some of the personality factors that may constitute a risk for developing a full-fledged psychopathic character organization.

The AAP analysis

John produced a valid, interpretable protocol. It was interpreted sequentially according to the primary dimensions of attachment operationalized in the AAP. The interpretation emphasizes both nomothetic (classification) and idiographic (person-specific) aspects of case formulation.

John's overall attachment classification is Dismissing. His protocol highlights several critical features associated with strong attempts to shut down attachment-related thoughts and feelings and focus on functional rather than reciprocal relationships. Stories involving characters alone typically focused on concrete action to manage attachment distress, in combination with defensive operations designed to neutralize activation of the attachment behavioral system. Two responses to the alone pictures provide a rich understanding of John's attachment representation and the projected alone self. The Windows story highlights John's dynamics[1]:

It's a sunny day... One sunny day, there's a girl, *the parents*	Deactivate
are at work, she's home alone. *She doesn't know what to*	Disconnect
do. She decides *she wants to maybe watch some TV, call*	
up a few friends, see what they're doing... She decides she	
wants to go out... She's out with her friends, *she sees the*	Agency: action
guy that she likes. The friends tell her that she should go	→ Deactivate
and say hi... She says she's too *shy.* Finally, the boy comes	Disconnect
over and introduces himself and asks if she wants to hang	
out... Her friends tell her she should go. She thinks about	
it for a minute and decides that she wants to hang out with	
him. They spend the day doing different things. *At the end*	Disconnect
of the day she says she had fun with him... And she would	
like to do it again sometime. He asks what she's doing	Deactivate
tomorrow, and she says "nothing." So they plan on getting	Agency: action,
together the next day. She goes home tells her parents	connect to
about it. They think it's great... Yeah, they think it's great,	attachment
and they encourage her. The end, I guess.	figures

A common theme for dismissing individuals when attachment needs are activated is to shift attention away from parents' inabilities to assuage attachment to functional connections to peers (affiliative-sociable system), often in peer romantic relationships (sexual system). We see this pattern play out in John's story. The parents' investment in their achievement leaves the self character (girl) confused about how to assuage attachment distress. Disconnected and confused, John entertains either deactivating his needs alone (watch TV) or drawing on his capacity to act and find friends. His affiliation with friends results in deactivation through the sexual system. The girl "sees a guy that she likes" and ends up spending the day with him. Upon returning home, she tells the parents about the experience and receives "encouragement" from them. The affiliative and romantic connectedness pattern is both activated and reinforced by John's attachment figures, who are at first absent. In the end, they encourage John's affiliative and romantic agency and social connections as compensatory strategies to manage attachment distress outside of the attachment system.

The Bench story embellishes on John's representational attachment dynamics.[2]

I walk into the *dressing room* and see... There's a girl sitting there crying. She looks upset... I *ask her what's wrong*... She says that... She says that she's been cut from *the team* ... I said it will be alright but she... *she can practice*... The next time <u>she can try out and make the team</u> (laughs)... *I say think about something that makes you happy, you can't dwell on the past, look forward, it will be alright*. The end, I guess. (think/feel?) Feeling? Sad... *angry* ...Yeah.	Deactivate Disconnect Deactivate Deactivate Agency: action Disconnect Deactivate Disconnect

A representation of deactivated selves dominates the narrative, the projected "girl" self and the insertion of "I" into the story as the central character. Developmentalists' theories of adolescents' multiple selves add to the interpretation of John's response juxtaposing the disavowed (person the adolescent dreads becoming) and ideal selves (the person the adolescent would like to be) (Chalk et al., 2005; Oyersman et al., 2015). The girl, the disavowed self, fails to meet performance standards, interpreted in the AAP as a form of deactivation that captures the negative evaluation that "leaks" when one fails to achieve and needs support. John's intervention as the ideal self demonstrates a kind of pseudo-empathy designed to keep the attachment behavioral system effectively neutralized; his idealized efforts at supporting his rejected self are somewhat formulaic in nature and gloss over attachment distress. Subtle devaluation of the other can be gleaned from using "...she can practice... The next time she can try out and make the team (laughs)." Thus, the impression is an idealized self characterized by superiority and invulnerability. This portrayal allows John to selectively deride and devalue aspects of himself that he perceives as vulnerable, similar to his behavior with his peer at school. As was the case in the Window story, distress is managed outside of the attachment system, probably suggesting that John generally shuts down attachment thoughts, feelings, and experiences. It is essential to point out here that dismissing individuals rarely admit to being angry. We might, therefore, suggest that John's internal conflict focused on anger is so profound that he was not able to exclude it from his narrative successfully.

The material presented in this response also evokes important questions regarding John's nature of gender relations. The scenario involves a failure to succeed in a competitive setting (girl not making the team). Following encouragement from John, the girl practices, tries out, and makes the team. The action depicted here is taken by a character who fails in competition, who eventually succeeds only after receiving support from John. The story thus features a juxtaposition between passivity and dependency on the one hand and the capacity to act that is conditional to receiving assistance provided by a male figure presented as being "in the lead." Stereotypical descriptions of gender roles, and those based on social scripts, are consistent with defensive attempts to decrease the potential for closeness between individuals and negate any possibility of the feared/disavowed self associated with the opposite gender interfering with the preservation of one's idealized self. John's use of the first person in some of the narratives, including Bench, is also consistent with the need to maintain an idealized representation of self. Implicit personality assessment methods are administered in a setting that requires that the subject ("I/self" – the examinee) engages in communication with an "Other" (the examiner) about a mediating object ("It" – the stimuli; Husain, 1996). In this context, it is not expected that the subject will use the assessment situation to talk about themselves directly – that is, to insert themselves into the story. This phenomenon seems to imply a blurring of the boundaries between the self and the stimuli. Such blurring may be the expression of a lack of awareness of the demarcation between self and external reality or a lack of consideration of the importance of such demarcation in interpersonal situations. In the latter case, the individual remains aware that the task of creating a narrative is not literally about them but may choose to insert themselves into the story to gratify a psychological need. The insertion is possibly linked to maintaining a grandiose self-image (O. Husain, personal communication, May 25, 2021). This element is consistent with John's behavior, which staff at the facility and his parents have described as entitled, egocentric, and self-centered.

John's dyadic responses feature relationship dynamics characterized by failed reciprocity between the characters. Processes of distancing any potential intimacy between attachment-caregiving dyads are also visible in the narratives, as exemplified by the inability of John to name the female character as the mother in his Ambulance story.[3]

A girl and her son... A woman and her son, sorry...They're at the hospital... The father has been in an accident. They...	
They're sitting there *hoping* for the best. They're seeing them	Disconnect
bringing him on a stretcher... They are *worried* ... They stay	Disconnect
all night. The next day *they get news* that he'll be alright...	Deactivate
They get to go and visit him. The end.	

John creates a narrative in which the boy's father had an accident, and what is implied to be the mother and her son are described as "hoping for the best." This defensive disconnection adds an element of uncertainty to the relationship with the father, creating a momentary smokescreen that prevents seeing the consequences of the father's accident. They eventually learn that the father "will be alright," and they visit him the next day. The story may easily give the impression of mutuality in the relationship between mother and son. However, the caregiver does not attempt to reassure or soothe the child's distress (worry) in a context of severe outcomes that could include the father's death. Thus, the parent figure and the child are described as both in a position of passive uncertainty. The source of their reassurance is deactivated and is described impersonally as "news" that manages that stress of uncertainty. When deactivated, John is ready to "reunite" with his attachment figure, avoiding lingering emotions. Interestingly, as for some of the other pictures, John initially identifies the adult character as a "girl," thus denying her identity as an attachment figure.

Clinical implications and outcome

The finding of a Dismissing attachment organization in John's case is not surprising since this particular attachment is prevalent in conduct-disordered adolescents (DeKlyen & Speltz, 2001). Beyond the attachment classification, however, case management must look at attachment organization and representational elements in the context of the youth's global functioning and life circumstances. In particular, attachment information must be translated into specific targets for interventions using a variety of modalities.

The clear emphasis on deactivating defenses in the context of attachment scenarios is essential to consider in light of strong concerns for possible emerging psychopathy in John's developmental trajectory. Callous-unemotional traits are a core dimension of juvenile psychopathy and can significantly impact the youth's potential for social adjustment and response to interventions (Frick et al., 2003). While John did not meet the formal criteria for psychopathy when assessed, this uncertainty regarding the diagnosis was primarily because he lacked an extensive history of serious offenses. However, it was noted that he displayed several characteristics associated with callous-unemotional traits, including pathological lying, tendency to manipulate, lack of remorse, lack of empathy, and failure to accept responsibility for his actions. Such traits are consistent with devaluation at the level of attachment (Adshead et al., 2012; Schimmenti et al., 2014). The presence of deactivation as a primary mechanism of defensive exclusion cannot be considered a diagnostic indicator of juvenile psychopathy, and most adolescent boys with a dismissing organization are not juvenile psychopaths. These features, however, can partially account for the emotional distancing and lack of empathy typically observed in psychopathic individuals (Meloy & Shiva, 2008).

From the perspective of case management, callous-unemotional, narcissistic, and dismissing features complicate the prognosis for successful rehabilitation, as they limit the potential for genuine collaboration in treatment. Individuals with these characteristics tend to show only surface compliance, pervasive oppositional and grandiose behaviors, and a lack of genuine investment in rehabilitative efforts. They may become worse as they get more exposure to therapeutic discourse, although the latter hypothesis has been questioned based on available research evidence (Hecht et al., 2018).

Recommendations in John's case were shared in separate meetings with the parents, John, and his case management team. His parents expressed feeling torn between their commitment to John and being genuinely afraid for their safety should he return home. They were very interested in learning about various "causes" for John's behaviors, particularly biological ones, and were disappointed when no definitive answer could be provided. John's tendency to avoid any kind of emotional intimacy with them in favor of peer relationships, his proclivity for action and his need to guard against any personal vulnerability were described to the parents. They agreed with these observations. They agreed that an eventual reintegration of John into the family home could only be envisioned in the context of a firm structure and clear contingencies in the event of misbehavior on his part. Measures were taken for the parents to liaise with community and health services in their community in the form of coaching and guidance in parenting practices.

John showed some curiosity regarding the findings, although he seemed primarily concerned with the impact that they would have on legal decisions about his sentence and reintegration into the community. As observed on the AAP, his attachment dynamics were described to him using specific elements from some of the stories as support. While he readily admitted actively maintaining a "larger than life" image of himself, he denied that this was a cover for underlying insecurity. He expressed wanting as little supervision as possible beyond his incarceration, as he was "missing out on his youth." At the time of the restitution session, he still had no clear plan on how he would be spending his time while in the community and what his future would be. The correctional staff felt that he was essentially "cruising through" his sentence, taking only marginal interest in rehabilitative activities and experiencing difficulties following directions. The need to maintain an impression of invulnerability and personal agency, as readily observed in the AAP protocol, meant that John was unable to allow himself to show any emotional fragility during his treatment. This inability conveyed an impression of emotional numbness that the therapeutic staff engaged in his care could not break through. Ultimately, it was recommended that weekly individual psychotherapy be attempted to see if he could respond to one-on-one contact on a stable basis. This recommendation was made based on AAP dyadic stories showing an acceptance of care, although from a functional perspective, not involving a secure, goal-corrected partnership.

In preparation for psychotherapeutic work with John, some consideration was given to ways to apply insights from the assessment of attachment to the formulation of strategies to facilitate meaningful change. In general, attachment-informed approaches to psychotherapy emphasize the modification of internal representations of relationships via a corrective emotional experience in the context of the client-therapist dynamic (Dales & Jerry, 2008; Holmes, 2017). Sustained and stable interaction patterns between therapist and client are intended to provide the latter with newer, more flexible, and adaptive templates for relationships, in the context of the client-therapist relationship being used as a secure base for exploration. In this context, the AAP attachment profile was essential in providing specific targets for therapeutic work with John.

John's overall dismissing organization is an important aspect of his functioning that can orient therapeutic strategies in his case. Dismissing adolescents, especially those at a more severe end of the deactivation spectrum (i.e., cannot tolerate conscious feelings of insecurity), typically experience difficulties recognizing a need for self-exploration and change. Strong defenses appear to effectively shut down the attachment behavioral system (Bowlby, 1980, 1982) to avoid feeling distressed, vulnerable, or insecure. Obtaining the client's trust and setting up a collaborative working alliance are thus primary goals at the beginning of therapy. Premature attempts at exploring emotions may be counter-productive and precipitate distancing and disengagement from the client (Dozier, 1990). It is essential to keep in mind that John's AAP representation of self revealed a firm reliance on action when he was alone (capacity to act) and functional unemotional interactions when he was in an attachment-caregiving dyad as his way to assuage attachment distress. Therefore, the therapist can expect that the initial distancing and disengagement mentioned above may likely take the form of behaviors that constitute attacks against the therapeutic setting, such as missing sessions, more or less direct insults and devaluation of the professional, and defensive use of humor (Gilliéron, 1987). This possibility is all the more substantial, given John's tendency to blur boundaries on multiple levels in the AAP.

Consequently, the therapist should ensure that the relationship with John is non-coercive, addresses concrete issues, and involve reasonable expectations in terms of finding and implementing solutions to problems in the institutional and family environment. In other words, as observed in his attachment narratives, John's propensity for acting and achievement could be capitalized on to co-create experiences of success and to learn in the therapeutic relationship. At the same time, testing boundaries and attempts at getting the therapist to engage in collusions should be met with firm interventions designed to reframe and make sense of these behaviors from a relational perspective.

John's AAP suggested a capacity to connect with others on a superficial and pragmatic level but little investment in terms of reciprocity and caregiving. It is possible that he will initially make a "good impression" on a therapist and will use the "right words" to convey that he has implemented significant changes since his incarceration. This dynamic was observed, for instance, in the Bench story, in which John created a "successful" outcome based on his capacity to act and social, gender-based dominance. This pattern is frequently observed in conduct-disordered individuals who also feature psychopathic characteristics (Meloy & Shiva, 2008). The therapist must go beyond superficial communications designed to influence others to target deeper internal states. With dismissing adolescents, this communication may initially involve putting affects into words in the hope that the need for emotional distancing may decrease over time. This decrease, in turn, may lead to a gradual opening to the exploration of an inner world to which John may have had no previous access (Dubois et al., 2013).

At the time of this writing, roughly four months following the feedback sessions with John and the custodial staff, a therapist still has not been found for him due to staff shortage. The staff at the institution were leaning toward recommending a transition into a less-secure supervised care facility to prepare John for potential reintegration into the community. However, they faced substantial resistance from the parents to John's return to the community in their vicinity. They voiced their concern that following the end of supervision orders, he would be left without guidance and seek the security he craves through antisocial misadventures and deviant peer affiliations.

Conclusion

This chapter illustrates the use of the AAP classification and coding material in the assessment and formulation of therapeutic objectives for conduct-disordered adolescents. The case of John, a 16-year-old inmate in a correctional facility, was presented. Key elements of John's attachment dynamics were highlighted using salient features of his AAP narratives. These elements included a Dismissing attachment pattern, focus on functional rather than reciprocal or synchronous relationships, deactivation as a primary defensive process, reliance on action rather than mentalizing activity as a method of managing attachment needs, and an emphasis on maintaining an idealized self-structure in order to protect against emotional vulnerability. These facets of John's functioning are consistent with conduct disorder, with primary psychopathy being a distinct possibility. Attachment information proved to be central to the formulation of therapeutic objectives for John beyond what is provided by conventional broadband personality assessment instruments. More specifically, it was recommended that given John's Dismissing attachment pattern, both behavioral management and individual psychotherapy be implemented to increase the likelihood of meaningful change. The hope is that by establishing a secure base with an experienced therapist, John would become gradually more open to exploring his emotions, including deep-seated needs for attachment and emotional closeness.

Notes

1 Italics = defenses; underline = capacity to act
2 Italics = defenses; underlined = capacity to act
3 Italics = defenses

References

Adshead, G., Brodrick, P., Preston, J., & Deshpande, M. (2012). Personality disorder in adolescence. *Advances in Psychiatric Treatment, 18*(2), 109–118. https://doi.org/10.1192/apt.bp.110.008623

Bowlby, J. (1979). The Bowlby-Ainsworth attachment theory. *Behavioral and Brain Sciences, 2*(4), 637–638. https://doi.org/10.1017/S0140525X00064955

Bowlby, J. (1980). *Attachment and loss: Vol. 3. Loss*. Basic Books.

Bowlby, J. (1982). *Attachment and loss: Vol. 1. Attachment*. Basic Books. (Original work published 1969)

Cardinale, E. M., Breeden, A. L., Robertson, E. L., Lozier, L. M., Vanmeter, J. W., & Marsh, A. A. (2018). Externalizing behavior severity in youths with callous-unemotional traits corresponds to patterns of amygdala activity and connectivity during judgments of causing fear. *Development and Psychopathology, 30*(1), 191–201. https://doi.org/10.1017/S0954579417000566

Chalk, L. M., Meara, N. M., Day, J D., & Davis, K. L. (2003). Occupational selves: Fears and aspirations of young college women. *Journal of Career Assessment, 13*(2), 188–203. https://doi.org/10.1177/1069072704273127

Dales, S., & Jerry, P. (2008). Attachment, affect regulation and mutual synchrony in adult psychotherapy. *American Journal of Psychotherapy, 62*(3), 283–312. https://doi.org/10.1176/appi.psychotherapy.2008.62.3.283

DeKlyen, M., & Speltz, M. L. (2001). Attachment and conduct disorder. In J. Hill & B. Maughan (Eds.), *Conduct disorders in childhood and adolescence* (pp. 320–345). Cambridge University Press.

Dozier, M. (1990). Attachment organization and treatment use for adults with serious psychopathological disorders. *Development and Psychopathology, 2*(1), 47–60. https://doi/10.1017/S0954579400000584

Dubois-Comtois, K., Cyr, C., Pascuzzo, K, Lessard, M. (2013) Attachment Theory in Clinical Work with Adolescents. *Journal of Child and Adolescent Behavior, 1*(3), https://doi.org10.4172/2375-4494.1000111.

Forth, A. E., Kosson, D. S., & Hare, R. D. (2003). *Hare psychopathy checklist: Youth Version*. Multi Health Systems.

Frick, P. J., Cornell, A. H., Bodin, S. D., Dane, H. E., Barry, C. T., & Loney, B. R. (2003). Callous-unemotional traits and developmental pathways to severe conduct problems. *Developmental Psychology, 39*(2), 246–260. https://doi.org/10.1037//0012-1649.39.2.246

Gambin, M., & Sharp, C. (2016). The differential relations between empathy and internalizing and externalizing symptoms in inpatient adolescents. *Child Psychiatry and Human Development, 47*(6), 966–974. https://doi.org/10.1007/s10578-016-0625-8

George, C., & West, M. (2020). *Adult attachment projective picture system: Protocol and classification scoring system* [Unpublished Manual], Mills College, CA.

George, C., & West, M. L. (2012). *The adult attachment projective picture system: Attachment theory and assessment in adults.* Guilford Press.

Gilliéron, E. (1987). Setting and motivation in brief psychotherapy. *Psychotherapy and Psychosomatics, 47*(2), 105–112. https://doi.org/ 10.1159/000288005.

Hecht, L. K., Latzman, R. D., & Lilienfeld, S. O. (2018). The psychological treatment of psychopathy. In D. David, S. J. Lynn, & G. H. Montgomery (Eds.), *Evidence-based psychotherapy* (pp. 271–298). John Wiley.

Holmes, J. (2017). Roots and routes to resilience and its role in psychotherapy: A selective, attachment-informed review. *Attachment and Human Development, 19*(4), 364–381. https://doi.org/10.1080/14616734.2017.1306087

Husain, O. (1996). Structure du fonctionnement d'un penser sans « je »: À propos du penser psychotique aux techniques projectives. *Psychologie Clinique et Projective, 2*(2), 219–244.

Meloy, J. R. (1992). *Violent attachments.* Jason Aronson.

Meloy, J. R., & Shiva, A. (2008). A psychoanalytic view of the psychopath. In A. Felthous & H. Sab (Eds.), *The international handbook of psychopathic disorders and the law* (pp. 335–346). John Wiley.

Mikulincer, M., & Shaver, P. R. (2012). An attachment perspective on psychopathology. *World Psychiatry, 11*(1), 11–15. https://doi.org/10.1016/j.wpsyc.2012.01.003

Oyersman, D., Destin, M., & Novin, S. (2015). The context sensitive future self: Possible selves motivate in context, not otherwise. *Self and Identity, 14(2),* 173–188. https://doi.org/10.1080/15298868.2014.965733

Pasalich, D. S., Dadds, M. R., Hawes, D. J., & Brennan, J. (2012). Attachment and callous-unemotional traits in children with early-onset conduct problems. *Journal of Child Psychology and Psychiatry, and Allied Disciplines, 53*(8), 838–845. https://doi.org/10.1111/j.1469-7610.2012.02544.x

Piccirillo, M. L., & Rodebaugh, T. L. (2019). Foundations of idiographic methods in psychology and applications for psychotherapy. *Clinical Psychology Review, 71,* 90–100. https://doi.org/10.1016/j.cpr.2019.01.002

Rosenstein, D. S., & Horowitz, H. A. (1996). Adolescent attachment and psychopathology. *Journal of Consulting and Clinical Psychology, 64*(2), 244–253. https://doi.org/10.1037//0022-006x.64.2.244

Schimmenti, A., Passanisi, A., Pace, U., Manzella, S., Di Carlo, G., & Caretti, V. (2014). The relationship between attachment and psychopathy: A study with a sample of violent offenders. *Current Psychology, 33*(3), 256–270. https://doi.org/10.1007/s12144-014-9211-z

Song, J.-H., Waller, R., Hyde, L. W., & Olson, S. L. (2016). Early callous-unemotional behavior, theory-of-mind, and a fearful/inhibited temperament predict externalizing problems in middle and late childhood. *Journal of Abnormal Child Psychology, 44*(6), 1205–1215. https://doi.org/10.1007/s10802-015-0099-3

Steiner, H., Remsing, L., & Work Group on Quality Issues. (2007). Practice parameter for the assessment and treatment of children and adolescents with oppositional defiant disorder. *Journal of the American Academy of Child* and Adolescent Psychiatry, 46(1), 126–141. https://doi.org/10.1097/01.chi.0000246060.62706.af

Taubner, S., White, L. O., Zimmermann, J., Fonagy, P., & Nolte, T. (2013). Attachment-related mentalization moderates the relationship between psychopathic traits and proactive aggression in adolescence. *Journal of Abnormal Child Psychology*, 41(6), 929–938. https://doi.org/10.1007/s10802-013-9736-x

Taubner, S., Zimmermann, L., Ramberg, A., & Schröder, P. (2016). Mentalization mediates the relationship between early maltreatment and potential for violence in adolescence. *Psychopathology*, 49(4), 236–246. https://doi.org/10.1159/000448053

van der Zouwen, M., Hoeve, M., Hendriks, A. M., Asscher, J. J., & Stams, G. J. (2018). The association between attachment and psychopathic traits. *Aggression and Violent Behavior*, 43, 45–55. https://doi.org/10.1016/j.avb.2018.09.002

Index

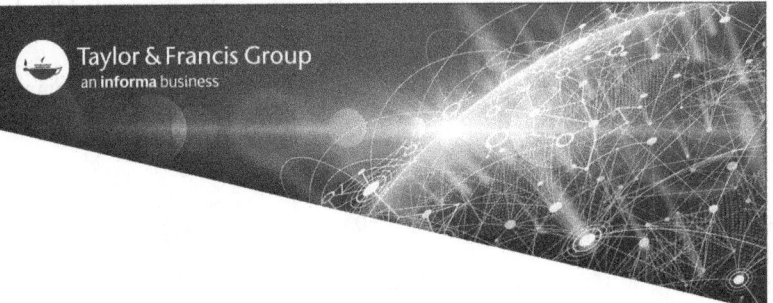
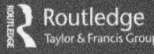
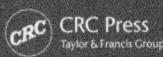